Collins

Lake District
Park Rangers
Favourite Walks

T0317898

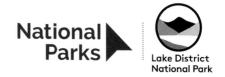

National Parks

Lake District
National Park

Published by Collins
An imprint of HarperCollins*Publishers*
Westerhill Road, Bishopbriggs, Glasgow G64 2QT
collins.reference@harpercollins.co.uk
www.harpercollins.co.uk

HarperCollins*Publishers*
1st Floor, Watermarque Building, Ringsend Road, Dublin 4, Ireland

Printed in Bosnia and Herzegovina

ISBN   978-0-00-843914-9   10 9 8 7 6 5 4 3 2 1

Contents

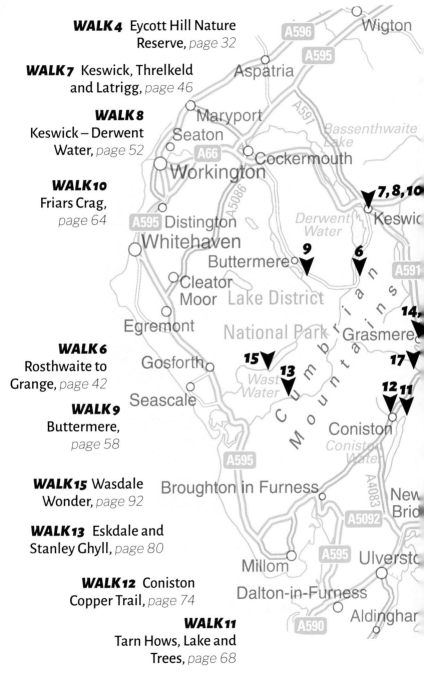

Wigton

A596

A595

Aspatria

Maryport

Seaton

A66

Bassenthwaite Lake

Workington

Cockermouth

A5086

Distington

A595

Whitehaven

Derwent Water

Keswick

7, 8, 10

Buttermere

9

6

A591

Cleator Moor

Lake District

Egremont

National Park

Cumbrian Mountains

Grasmere

14,

Gosforth

15

13

17

Wast Water

Seascale

12 11

Coniston

Coniston Water

A595

Broughton in Furness

New Bri

A5092

Millom

A595

Ulversto

Dalton-in-Furness

A590

Aldinghar

WALK
LOCATIONS

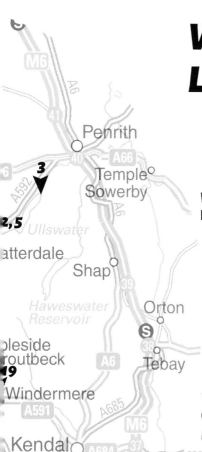

▼ Recommended starting point for each route – refer to individual walk instructions for more details.

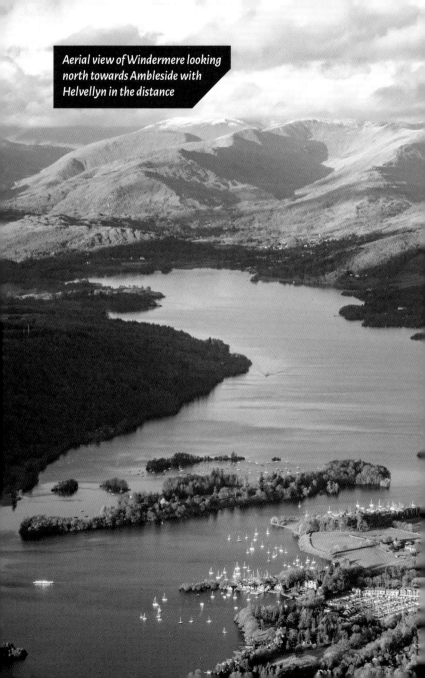

Aerial view of Windermere looking north towards Ambleside with Helvellyn in the distance

Introduction

The Lake District National Park is the largest of the National Parks in England and Wales, covering 912 square miles (2362 sq km) of countryside. It was designated as a National Park in 1951 – the second National Park to be designated this way (after the Peak District which had been designated one month earlier) – and kept its original boundaries until 2016 when it was extended slightly to incorporate some hills in the etreme eastern edge.

In many countries of the world National Parks are areas of wilderness hardly influenced by man, however there is no true wilderness left in England. The 'natural' beauty of the landscape reflects the pattern of husbandry, with many individuals and organisations owning and making a living from the land. A British National Park is a defined area of unspoilt countryside, usually with some wild, if not wilderness, country, which is specially protected from unsuitable development; public access for its enjoyment is secured, and due regard made for the needs of the local community. The Lake District is an excellent example of such an place.

In 1969 England's first National Park Visitor Centre was set up at Brockhole in Windermere and it remains an excellent starting point for exploration of the National Park. The National Trust and the Lake District National Park Authority work closely with other large landowners, the Forestry Commission and the Water Authority, to provide protected public access unrivalled anywhere else in Britain. It is indeed as Wordsworth said 'a sort of national property' for those 'with eyes to perceive and hearts to enjoy'

What is seen now in the Lake District still reads historically from north to south. The mountains and hills of Skiddaw Slates which lie in a curving band, from the north to the west, are covered by carboniferous limestones and sandstones nearer the coast, and reappear to the south-west at Black Combe. Because much of this material is shaley and craggy outcrops seldom occur, the fells have angular outlines. Skiddaw itself (3054 ft/931 m) and its neighbour Blencathra (2847 ft/868 m), are good examples. The fells to the west of Derwentwater, Causey Pike and Grisedale Pike, are of the same material, and the rock is also very evident in the fells on the east side of Buttermere, to the north and west around Crummock Water and Loweswater as well as the northern end of Ennerdale Water. There is good soil depth on these rock forms which allows trees and heather to grow naturally.

In the central Lake District, roughly north-east to south-west are the high craggy fells of the Scafells, Great Gable, the Borrowdale fells, as well as Coniston Old Man in the south-west through the Langdales and Bowfell; and eastwards through Helvellyn to High Street. Here, the shallow acidic soils do not support a rich vegetation. The alpine plants are found mainly where springs leach the minerals to the surface. The deeper soils are often covered in bracken, very beautifully coloured in autumn, but useless to the hill farmers' sheep.

From another type of rock, formed from fine volcanic sediments in water, comes the famous green slate, still quarried and much in demand for its wearing and decorative qualities. It is used for the facings of prestigious buildings. The Honister Slate Mines on the Honister Pass closed in 1986 after three centuries of production. However, it reopened in 1997 as a working slate mine and has become one of the leading attractions in the Lake District.

In the south of the Lake District the soft slates and mudstones produce an acid soil in which trees and forests find root and regenerate quite readily. The typical scenery, much in evidence around Windermere, consists of rounded hills, often with a good deal of tree cover. The Forestry Commission's largest forest, at Grizedale is also in this area.

Due to the huge variety of landscapes to be found in a relatively small area, there are diverse habitats for flora and fauna to thrive. Many different types of grassland, upland heath and mires are designated areas of habitat conservation and protected plant species include juniper and the slender green feather-moss. There are several National Nature Reserves, over 100 Sites of Special Scientific Interest and many other conservation areas.

Old fashioned hay meadows are rich in various species of wild flowers and butterflies, while Red grouse can be regularly seen on the heather and sphagnum moss of the moorlands. The National Park is also home to some of the country's rarest creatures. Derwent Water is the only place in the country where you can find the vendace – the UK's rarest freshwater fish – while the schelly is still to be found in Brothers Water, Haweswater, Red Tarn and Ullswater. Ospreys still return every year to Bassenthwaite Lake (they first nested there in 2001) and across large parts of the park you can still catch a glimpse of a red squirrel.

With such a diverse landscape there is a huge variety of terrain for walkers of any age and ability. There is something for everyone – low-level lakeside walks, exposed ridge walks, strolls through forests and thrilling mountain walks. Even at the height of summer when the towns and the more popular destinations are teeming with tourists it is still possible to get away from it all and find secluded areas where the magnificent countryside can be enjoyed in relative solitude.

Always keep in mind that the weather can change rapidly and a lovely summer's day can quickly change to a torrential downpour especially at higher altitudes. Scafell Pike at 3,209 ft (978 m) is the highest point in England and at 10½ miles (16.5km) in length Windermere is its longest lake. Wind that can seem pretty tame in the shelter of a small town or village can feel quite different at the top of a hill or in the middle of an expanse of water.

Walking is a pastime which can fulfil the needs of everyone. You can adapt it to suit your own preferences and it is one of the healthiest of activities. This guide is for those who just want to walk a few miles. It really doesn't take long to find yourself in some lovely countryside in the Lake District National Park.

Getting around

The Lake District National Park is well connected by road and rail with the rest of the country. The West Coast mainline runs to the east of the National Park, connecting Oxenholme, Penrith and Carlisle with London and Glasgow. A direct train runs from Manchester to Windermere. Local trains call at Kendal, Staveley and Windermere. There is also a route along the Cumbrian coastline between Carlisle and Barrow-in-Furness, Lancaster and Preston. For more details contact National Rail enquiries: 03457 484950 **www.nationalrail.co.uk**

For drivers coming from any distance, the main entry to the Lake District is usually via the M6 which also runs down the eastern edge of the National Park. All junctions between 36 in the south to 44 in the north offer access to the park, with the main ones being 37 for Kendal and Windermere and 40 for Keswick and Ullswater. Much of the National Park is accessible by road but keep in mind that away from the main routes, roads can get very narrow, steep and sat navs don't always work too well. Parking can also be expensive and spaces in car parks can fill by mid morning even in quieter months.

National Express (0871 781 8181 **www.nationalexpress.com**) run coaches from all over the country to Carlisle and Penrith just outside the National Park. Once in the area, local bus services cross the Lake District with dayrider and explorer tickets giving unlimited travel, but you'll want to check their regularity ahead of time.

Many of the walks in the book are close to bigger towns and this is so that you can start your walk from a bus or train station. Otherwise cycling is still an excellent way of getting about. For more information on cycling in the Lake District National Park: **https://www.lakedistrict.gov.uk/visiting/things-to-do/cycling**

Protecting the countryside

The Lake District National Park Authority wants everyone to enjoy their visit and to help keep the area a special place. You can do this by following the Countryside Code.

RESPECT EVERYONE

- Be considerate to those living in, working in and enjoying the countryside.
- Leave gates and property as you find them.
- Do not block access to gateways or driveways when parking.
- Be nice, say hello, share the space.
- Follow local signs and keep to marked paths unless wider access is available.

PROTECT THE NATURAL ENVIRONMENT

- Take your litter home – leave no trace of your visit.
- Take care with BBQs and do not light fires.
- Always keep your dogs under control and in sight.
- Dog poo – bag it and bin it in any public waste bin.
- Care for nature – do not cause damage or disturbance.

ENJOY THE OUTDOORS

- Check your route and local conditions.
- Plan your adventure – know what to expect and what you can do.
- Enjoy your visit, have fun, make a memory.

It's pretty easy to act responsibly when out walking. Simply take care not to disturb wild animals and sensitive habitats. Don't take things away like stones or wild flowers, and don't leave anything behind that you shouldn't. Walkers should take extra care to stick to paths where they can especially during nesting seasons (typically late spring to early summer). For more details about the countryside code check out: **https://www.lakedistrict.gov.uk/visiting/countryside-code**

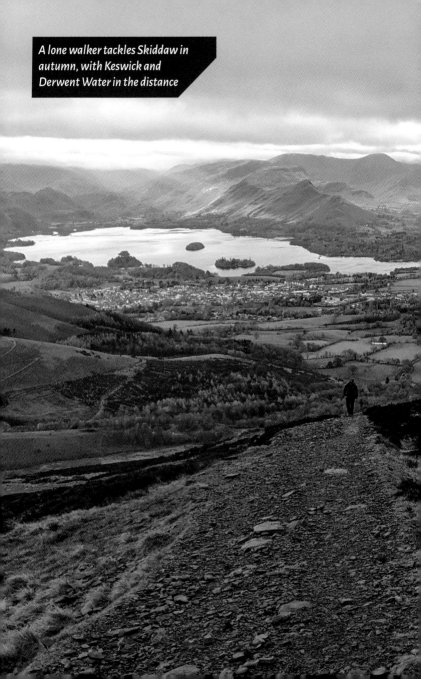

A lone walker tackles Skiddaw in autumn, with Keswick and Derwent Water in the distance

Walking tips & guidance

Safety

Walking will be safe and enjoyable provided a few simple rules are followed:

- Make sure you are fit enough to complete the walk.

- Always try to let others know where you intend to go.

- Take care around cliff edges and keep an eye on the tide.

- Wear sensible clothes and suitable footwear.

- Take ample water and food.

- Take a map or guide.

- Always allow plenty of time for the walk and be aware of when it will get dark.

- Walk at a steady pace. A zigzag route is usually a more comfortable way of negotiating a slope. Avoid going directly downhill as it's easier to lose control and may also cause erosion to the hillside.

- When walking on country roads, walk on the right-hand side facing the oncoming traffic, unless approaching a blind bend when you should cross over to the left so as to be seen from both directions.

- Try not to dislodge stones on high edges or slopes.

- If the weather changes unexpectedly and visibility becomes poor, don't panic, but try to remember the last certain feature you passed and work out your route from that point on the map. Be sure of your route before continuing.

Unfortunately, accidents can happen even on easy walks. If you're with someone who has an accident or can't continue, you should:

- Make sure the injured person is sheltered from further injury, although you should never move anyone with a head, neck or back injury.

- If you have a phone with a signal, call for help.

- If you can't get a signal and have to leave the injured person to go for help, try to leave a note saying what has happened and what first aid you have tried. Make sure you know the exact location so you can give accurate directions to the emergency services. When you reach a telephone call 999 and ask for the Police and Mountain Rescue.

Equipment

The equipment you will need depends on several factors, such as the type of activity planned, the time of year, and the weather likely to be encountered.

Clothing should be adequate for the day. In summer, remember sun screen, especially for your head and neck. Wear light woollen socks and lightweight boots or strong shoes. Even on hot days take an extra layer and waterproofs in your rucksack, just in case. Winter wear is a much more serious affair. Remember that once the body starts to lose heat, it becomes much less efficient. Jeans are particularly unsuitable for winter walking.

When considering waterproof clothing, it pays to buy the best you can afford. Make sure that the jacket is loose-fitting, windproof and has a generous hood. Waterproof overtrousers will not only offer protection against the rain, but they are also windproof. Clothing described as 'showerproof' will not keep you dry in heavy rain, and those made from rubberized or plastic materials can be heavy to carry and will trap moisture on the inside. Your rucksack should have wide, padded carrying straps for comfort.

It is important to wear boots that fit well or shoes with a good moulded sole – blisters can ruin any walk! Woollen socks are much more comfortable than any other fibre. Your clothes should be comfortable and not likely to catch on twigs and bushes.

It is important to carry a compass and a map or guide. A small first aid kit is also useful for treating cuts and other small injuries.

Finally, take a bottle of water and enough food to keep you going.

Public rights of way
Right of way means that anyone may walk freely on a defined footpath or ride a horse or bicycle along a public bridleway. In 1949, the National Parks and Access to the Countryside Act tidied up the law covering rights of way. Following public consultation, maps were drawn up by the Countryside Authorities of England and Wales to show all rights of way. Copies of these maps are available for public inspection and are invaluable when trying to resolve doubts over little-used footpaths. Once on the map, the right of way is irrefutable.

Any obstructions to a right of way should be reported to the local Highways Authority.

In England and Wales rights of way fall into three main categories:

- Public footpaths – for walkers only.

- Bridleways – for passage on foot, horseback or bicycle.

- Byways – for all the above and for motorized vehicles.

Free access to footpaths and bridleways does mean that certain guidelines should be followed as a courtesy to those who live and work in the area. For example, you should only sit down to picnic where it does not interfere with other walkers or the landowner. All gates must be kept closed to prevent stock from straying and dogs must be kept under close control – usually this is interpreted as meaning that they should be kept on a lead. Motorised vehicles must not be driven along a public footpath or bridleway without the landowner's consent.

A farmer may put a docile mature beef bull with a herd of cows or heifers, in a field crossed by a public footpath. Beef bulls such as Herefords (usually brown / red in colour) are unlikely to be upset by passers-by but dairy bulls, like the black-and-white Friesian, can be dangerous by nature. It is, therefore, illegal for a farmer to let a dairy bull roam loose in a field open to public access.

The Countryside and Rights of Way Act 2000 allows access on foot to areas of legally defined 'open country' – mountain, moor, downland, heath and registered common land. It does not allow freedom to walk everywhere. It also increases protection for Sites of Special Scientific Interest, improves wildlife enforcement legislation and allows for better management of Areas of Outstanding Natural Beauty.

How to use this book

Each of the walks in this guide are set out in a similar way. They are all introduced with a simple locator map followed by a brief description of the area, its geography and history, and some notes on things you will encounter on your walk.

Near the start of each section there is a panel of information outlining the distance of the walk, the time it is expected to take and briefly describing the path conditions or the terrain you will encounter. A suggested starting point, along with grid reference is shown, as is the nearest postcode – although in rural locations postcodes can cover a large area and are therefore only a rough guide for sat nav users. It is always sensible to take a reference map with you, and the relevant OS Explorer map is also listed.

The major part of each section is taken up with a plan for each walk and detailed point by point, description of our recommended route, along with navigational tips and points of interest.

Here is a description of the main symbols on the route maps:

Motorway	Railway station	Contour height (m)
Trunk/primary road	Bus station/stop	Walk route
Secondary road	Car park	Optional route
Tertiary road	Castle	Route instruction
Residential/unclassified road	Church	Open land
Service road	Lighthouse	Parks/sports grounds
Track	Interesting feature	Urban area
Pedestrian/bridleway/cycleway	Tourist information	Woodland
Footway/path	Cafe	Nature reserve
Railway	Pub	Wetland
Rivers/coast	Toilets	Lakes

WALK 1
Howtown to Patterdale

The perfect combination of cruise and walk, this route is an opportunity to experience the magic of Ullswater from the water, lakeshore and fellside. Alfred Wainwright, famous for his Guides to the Fells, described this as "the most beautiful and rewarding walk in Lakeland."

The path climbs out of Howtown to reveal stunning views north towards Dunmallard Hill and the Pennines beyond. It then winds through ancient Hallinhag woodland before dipping down to the lakeshore. In the wood discover three Poetry Stones, inscribed with words from the poems of Kathleen Raine who lived in nearby Martindale in the 1940s.

After crossing the beck in Sandwick and passing the waterfalls of Scalehow Force, a glance up to the crags may reveal a peregrine in flight or, in winter, the silhouette of a red deer on the skyline. Red squirrels can be seen in the woods or running along the walls.

From Silver Point there are magnificent views across the lake to the hanging valley of Glencoyne and the 17th century farmhouse below. Beyond, the foothills of Helvellyn rise majestically behind the village of Glenridding, once home to the largest lead mine in the country, now better known as the home of the Ullswater Steamers. Their flagship, "Lady of the Lake" is believed to be the oldest working passenger vessel in the world.

This walk is a section of the very popular Ullswater Way 20-mile walking route which circumnavigates Ullswater. The route is well waymarked and can easily be broken up into four distinct sections linking with the steamers or local bus service.

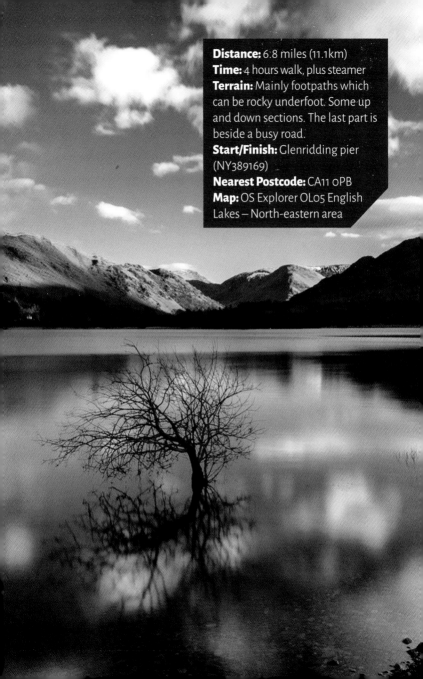

Distance: 6.8 miles (11.1km)
Time: 4 hours walk, plus steamer
Terrain: Mainly footpaths which can be rocky underfoot. Some up and down sections. The last part is beside a busy road.
Start/Finish: Glenridding pier (NY389169)
Nearest Postcode: CA11 0PB
Map: OS Explorer OL05 English Lakes – North-eastern area

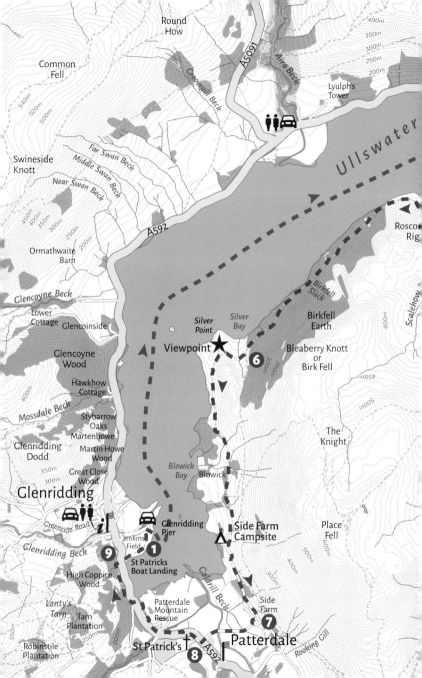

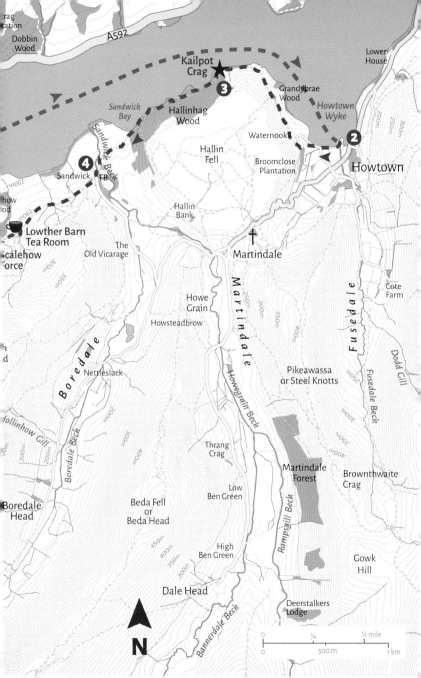

Parking can be expensive and quickly fills during busy periods, so you may want to arrive at the starting point by bus. Buses run from Penrith and Penrith Railway Station to Pooley Bridge, Glenridding and Patterdale, with open top buses in summer on service 508, operated by Stagecoach. In the summer they continue over Kirkstone pass to link with Windermere and Bowness. More details from travelline **www.traveline.org.uk.** Steamers run from Glenridding or Pooley Bridge to Howtown. Details of timetable and fares can be found at **https://www.ullswater-steamers.co.uk/**

Parking is available in Glenridding, note there is no public parking in Howtown.

1 At Glenridding Pier board the "steamer" for Howtown and enjoy the magnificent lake and mountain scenery.

2 Disembark at Howtown Pier, at the end of which you bear right over a bridge and then follow the path along the lakeshore to a gate leading out onto a road. Head along the road for about 50 m, then left through a gate onto a path signed to Patterdale/ Sandwick. This takes you up some steps to another gate in a wall. Through this go right and follow the clear path above the SW side of Howtown Bay to the view point at Kialpot Crag.

3 Go down through the rocks and along the shore to the gate into Hallinhag Wood. Follow the path through the woods parallel to the shore, watching out for the sign for the Poetry Stones. Emerge at a gate and steps at Sandwick Bay. Here the path bears slightly left away from the lake and crosses gated fields to a bridge over the Sandwick Beck to a road.

4 Go left up the road for about 50 m then take a signed path on the right (to Patterdale). Follow along with a wall on your right until you reach Lowther Barn Café. Just beyond there is a stream crossing where you get views of Scalehow Force.

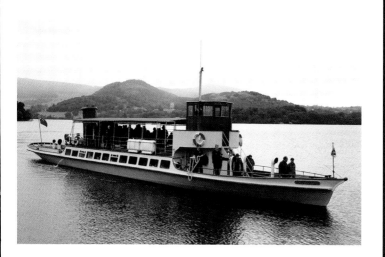

5 Continue along the clear path bearing right (NW) dropping down to the shore again. This undulating path continues to a viewpoint above the lake and emerges from the trees at Silver Bay.

6 At a path junction keep right along the path, initially on the level. You'll pass the Artists' Seat (an Ullswater Way feature), then Side Farm campsite and on to the gate at the yard to Side Farm.

7 Turn right between a barn and the farmhouse and go straight ahead on the track from the farm, crossing Goldrill Beck and out to the A592 road in Patterdale.

8 Turn right, keeping along the roadside path passing Patterdale Church and the Mountain Rescue Centre to Glenridding and St Patrick's Boatyard (this section involves crossing the A592 four times).

9 Go through the gate into the boatyard and ahead on the shoreline path in Jenkin's Field back to Glenridding Pier.

WALK 2
Aira Force and Glenridding

Magnificent lake views, a picturesque waterfall and the chance to walk in Wordsworth's footsteps, this short walk is packed with interest.

At Aira Force, winding paths climb through the forest to reveal the 20 m waterfall, at its best after heavy rain.

Leaving Aira Tea Room, the route parallels the shore of Ullswater through the wood pasture of Glencoyne Park with its wonderful ancient trees, any fallen branches left to decay naturally, providing habitats for wildlife. It was along this shore that the Wordsworths were walking when Dorothy noticed the dancing daffodils that she described in her diary and which inspired William to write his famous poem.

Glencoyne Farm, nestled behind its hay meadows, dates back to 1629 and has characteristic step gables and circular chimneys. Amongst the grazing sheep look out for Herdwicks, the typical grey-fleeced sheep of the Lake District, their lambs completely black.

The final section of the walk hugs the shore, providing beautiful views through the trees to the lake and its islands. It was here that Charles Darwin strolled with his wife and daughter when on holiday at Glenridding House in 1881.

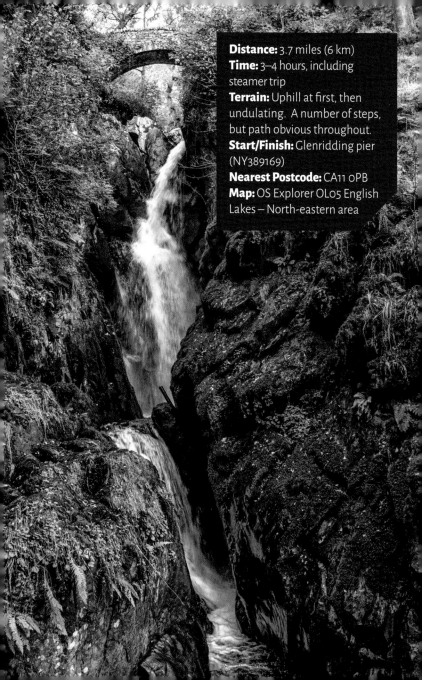

Distance: 3.7 miles (6 km)
Time: 3–4 hours, including steamer trip
Terrain: Uphill at first, then undulating. A number of steps, but path obvious throughout.
Start/Finish: Glenridding pier (NY389169)
Nearest Postcode: CA11 0PB
Map: OS Explorer OL05 English Lakes – North-eastern area

1 At Glenridding Pier, take boat to Aira Force enjoying wonderful scenery.

2 From Aira pier walk up to the road, cross straight over and take path around tea-room. Soon bear left to avoid car park. Continue to "The Glade" then keeping right down to a wooden bridge over the stream and up steps. At a prominent spruce tree take a path to the right uphill, then after 50 m bear left. In another 50 m climb more steps. Keep on the path to the left until the bridge at the top of the waterfall.

3 Cross bridge, head up more steps and left down to top of more steps. Go left down the steps (over 100) to a view point at the bottom of waterfall. Continue over the bridge and follow the path back to the spruce tree, "The Glade" and the tea room.

4 From the tea-room gate, go right and carefully cross A5091 to join a path going SW. This leads to a stone tree-fold structure. Continuing, the path crosses 4 bridges, then 50 m further on a path on the left goes down to a green gate. This gives access to A592 which is crossed to the lakeside wood – the home of Wordsworth's daffodils.

5 If you have a GPS you should be at NY388191. Return to main track heading left to Glencoyne car park. The path traverses the car park and continues south. After about 400 m, cross the A592 to path continuation on lakeside. Follow the path to top of hill and divert left for 10 m for a lake view. Continue on the path to meet the road opposite Hawkhow. Here it is necessary to walk along the road (keep on lake side) under Stybarrow Crag. The shore path resumes after 200 m. It soon goes up steps to a viewpoint, then down again and continues on to more steps up to another viewpoint.

6 Walk to the road and go left on the pavement through Glenridding village, over the beck and take the road on the left back to Glenridding Pier.

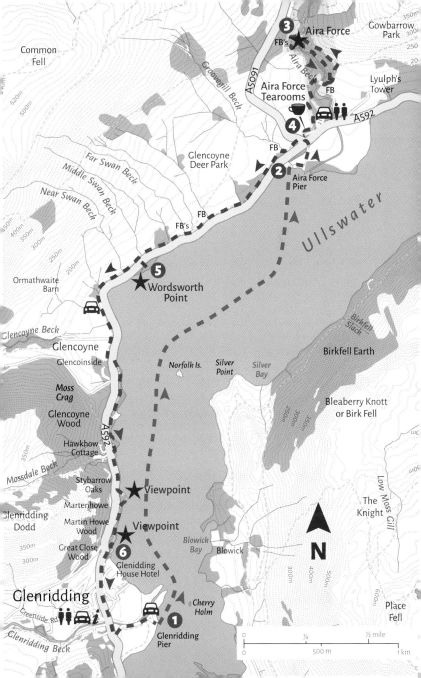

3 Aira Force

Gowbarrow Park

FB's

Common Fell

520m

500m

Groovegill Beck

A5091

Aira Beck

Aira Force Tearooms

FB

Lyulph's Tower

4

A592

350m

300m

250m

200

Far Swan Beck

Middle Swan Beck

Near Swan Beck

Glencoyne Deer Park

FB

2

Aira Force Pier

Ullswater

400m

350m

250m

FB

150m

FB's

Ormathwaite Barn

200m

5

★ Wordsworth Point

Birkfell Slack

Glencoyne Beck

Glencoyne

Glencoinside

Norfolk Is.

Silver Point

Silver Bay

350m

250m

Birkfell Earth

Moss Crag

Glencoyne Wood

A592

Bleaberry Knott or Birk Fell

350m

Hawkhow Cottage

Mossdale Beck

Stybarrow Oaks

★ Viewpoint

Low Moss Gill

300m

400m

500m

600m

Glenridding Dodd

Martenhowe

Martin Howe Wood

★ Viewpoint

The Knight

Great Close Wood

6

Glenidding House Hotel

N

Glenridding

Creenside Rd

Blowick Bay

Blowick

Place Fell

Glenridding Beck

1

Glenridding Pier

Cherry Holm

0 ¼ ½ mile

0 500 m 1 km

WALK 3
Dalemain Loop

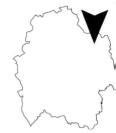

A walk back in time at the head of the lake.

From Dunmallard Hill, with an Iron Age fort on its summit, the route crosses open pasture, then a section of road walking, to reach the historic village of Dacre. Mystery surrounds the four bear statues to be found in the graveyard of St. Andrew's church and the church itself probably stands on the site of a monastery which was mentioned in the writing of Venerable Bede in AD 731. The Church has interesting windows and a Lady Anne Clifford key.

From the church the route then passes Dacre Castle, which is a Pele tower with a moat and walls seven feet thick and 66 feet high. It was built in the 14th century for protection against the marauding Scots – the boarders Reivers.

From Dacre the route follows a wide track to arrive at Dalemain and an opportunity to pause for refreshments in the Medieval Hall or courtyard before admiring its impressive Georgian façade. Guided tours are normally available.

The final stretch follows the River Eamont back to Pooley Bridge where the fish (a Schelly) on top of the cross reminds us that this was once a thriving fishing village. The Schelly is a fresh water fish of the salmon family, endemic to four lakes in the Lake District, including Ullswater.

❶ Leaving the village, cross the new bridge and pass through a gate into the wood. Go right but take left fork after 20 m going fairly steeply uphill through the woods. After 350 m

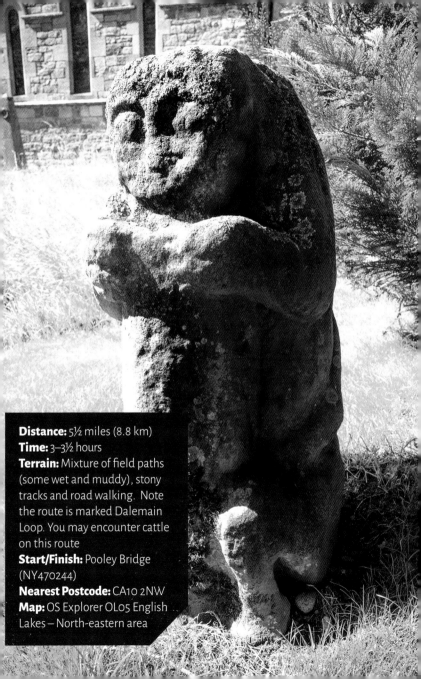

Distance: 5½ miles (8.8 km)
Time: 3–3½ hours
Terrain: Mixture of field paths
(some wet and muddy), stony
tracks and road walking. Note
the route is marked Dalemain
Loop. You may encounter cattle
on this route
Start/Finish: Pooley Bridge
(NY470244)
Nearest Postcode: CA10 2NW
Map: OS Explorer OL05 English
Lakes – North-eastern area

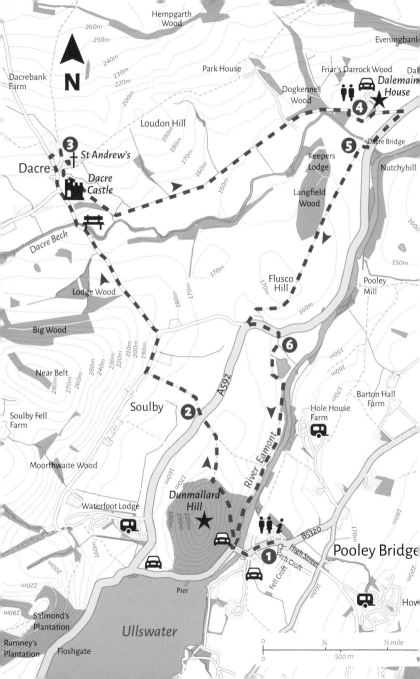

Hempgarth Wood

Eveningbank

Dacrebank Farm

Park House

Friar's Darrock Wood

Da

Dalemain House

Dogkennel Wood

Loudon Hill

260m
250m
240m
230m
220m
200m
190m
180m
170m
160m
150m

3 St Andrew's

Dacre

Dacre Castle

Keepers Lodge

Dacre Bridge

5

Nutchyhill

Langfield Wood

160m

Dacre Beck

150m

170m

Lodge Wood

170m
170m
180m

Flusco Hill

170m

160m

Pooley Mill

Big Wood

Near Belt

280m
270m
260m
250m
240m
230m
220m
210m
200m
190m

6

A592

Soulby

2

Soulby Fell Farm

Barton Hall Farm

Hole House Farm

Moorthwaite Wood

160m
170m

Waterfoot Lodge

Dunmallard Hill

180m
200m
220m

River Eamont

Pooley Bridge

B5320

High Street

1

Fell Croft

Church Croft

Pier

Salmond's Plantation

160m

170m

180m

How

Ullswater

Rumney's Plantation

Floshgate

0   ¼   ½ mile

500 m

where the path swings to the left, go right through a gate, then continue across 2 fields passing through 2 more gates. Turn left immediately after the 2nd gate along the boundary down to A592.

2 Cross directly over to the bridleway in field opposite walking up to Soulby road with fence on the left (Note - there may be cows in these fields). Turn right along the road to T junction and turn left on road. Walk for 800 m to Dacre Bridge (wide verges here) and up into the village. Ignore signed track on the right and go on another 10 m to the road going half right to the church gate.

3 The church contains many items of interest while the Dacre Bear statues are in the graveyard. Leave the grounds by the gate in the south wall, turn right on path to join track going left past Dacre Castle. Keep left at a fork and carry on for almost 2 km to Dalemain House.

4 Just before Dalemain courtyard, in a field on the left, fallow deer are often seen. Leave the courtyard under an arch and follow the road to the entrance from A592. Turn right and walk down the verge for 250 m to a bridge and stile into a field on the right.

5 Head uphill keeping the woods to your right. At the top of the hill head directly towards Dunmallard Hill, following a track through 2 gates. Just after the 2nd gate ignore a track down to a gate as this is not a public Right of Way (note there may be sheep in these fields so keep dogs on lead). Pass through a gate and over a stone bridge to a stone stile which brings you out at the A592 / Dacre Road junction. Go left down the A592 using verge on right for 150 m to a gate.

6 Go right through a gate then follow path close to the fence on left over 2 plank bridges to a gate on the left. Pass through the gate and continue for 50 m, skirting a large pond down to another gate where the path goes right through the gate. Follow this riverside path through 5 gates back to the new bridge and left into Pooley Bridge.

WALK 4

Eycott Hill Nature Reserve

A quiet gem of a walk for nature lovers with the added benefits of stunning views of Blencathra and the northern fells combined with interesting archaeology and geology.

For centuries the land at Eycott Hill was owned by the Dukes of Norfolk. It went on the market in 2012 and was bought by the Esmee Fairbairn Foundation who kept it while the Cumbria Wildlife Trust raised the funds to buy the 530 acres in 2015 and turn it into a Nature Reserve.

A large area of the reserve is covered with andesite – a volcanic rock formed around 450 million years ago when the whole of the central Lake District was subjected to volcanic upheaval. 20 separate lava flows poured over the area causing mounds and furrows as each flow cooled and settled. Over the millennia the furrows have filled with water and peat, forming bogs which are ideal for wetland habitats.

Depending on the time of the year you visit, you will be rewarded by walking in the flower rich hay meadow or strolling by bog loving plants and a whole range of flowers that enjoy this upland habitat.

Over the centuries, tenant farmers had the right to cut peat which was usually burned as fuel. Over 20 sites of archaeological interest have been noted, probably from the 1700's to 1800's. These are a mixture of banks, animal enclosures and trackways probably indicating an attempt to farm the land.

Since buying the site, Cumbria Wildlife Trust has greatly improved the reserve. A well planned 5 year project has created a visitor

Distance: 2½ miles (4.1 km)   **Time:** 2–2½ hours
Terrain: Undulating and mostly over wet ground. Do not attempt to take short cuts away from the marked route as this could result in sinking into deep mire. Rare breed cattle roam freely over Eycott Hill. These are typically Belted Galloway which are very docile and ignore walkers.
Start/Finish: Cumbria Wildlife Trust car park (NY393300)
Nearest Postcode: CA11 0XD
Map: OS Explorer OL05 English Lakes – North-eastern area

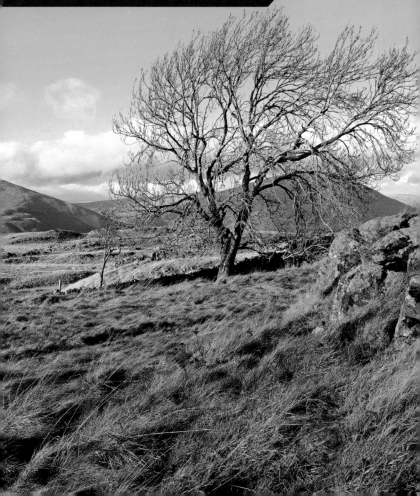

car park with visitor interpretation boards, well drained paths and boardwalks over wet areas. Trees and hedges have been planted and wildlife encouraged. The introduction of hardy Belted Galloway cattle has helped to break up the soil.

If you are looking for a quiet walk in nature, this is the walk for you.

1 Exit the car park by the gate onto a track going SW alongside a wall. At the bottom of the field turn right just before a gate. After 50 m, ignore another gate and bridge on the left but continue ahead to a field gate. Go through this turn left and continue through two more gates into a meadow. Walk up the slope (fence on left) to a gateway and go left into adjacent meadow. Now bear right diagonally up the slope to the exit gate in the top left corner. Just through the gate is a circular stone viewpoint.

2 Head south on the track with the wall on your right until you reach a gate.

3 Go through the gate and turn right, a path heads NW (marked with posts) over a hillock and down to a boardwalk over a mire. A second boardwalk is soon reached. The path then goes SW but veers left (to SE) and to a stream crossing, before continuing along the side of a prominent crag with a single tree on top.

4 After 2 hillocks the path turns abruptly right (NW) and soon climbs up to the rocky summit of Eycott Hill with wonderful all-round views.

5 Re-trace your steps (being aware of the sharp bend near the rock with single tree), over boardwalks back to gate in wall at **3**.

6 Go through the gate and ahead on broad green track (ignore fence posts – these are not markers). Approaching a line of trees and a fence, path swings to the right and goes to the gate into the field below car park. Through the gate go ahead to the car park.

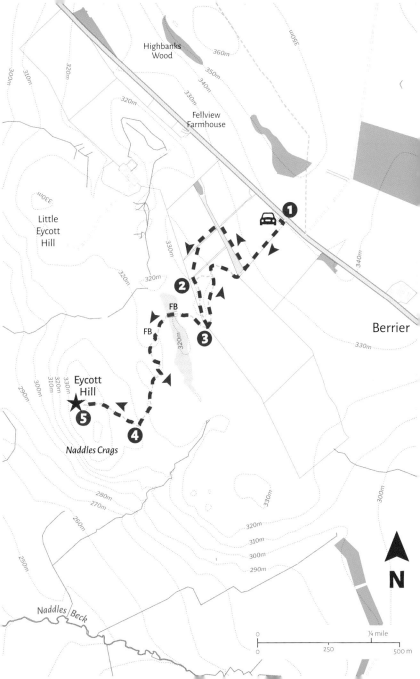

Highbanks
Wood

360m
350m
340m
330m
350m

Fellview
Farmhouse

320m

Little
Eycott
Hill

330m

330m

320m
320m

340m

330m

1

2

FB

FB

3

320m

Eycott
Hill

290m
300m
310m
320m
330m

5

4

Naddles Crags

Berrier

330m

280m
270m
260m

320m
310m
300m
290m

330m

300m

250m

Naddles Beck

N

0   ¼ mile
0   250   500 m

WALK 5
Glenridding and Lanty's Tarn

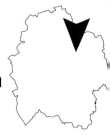

This interesting walk combines both the history of the village of Glenridding with breathtaking views over Ullswater.

Glenridding is the site of what was once the most important lead mine in the country. Mining probably began here in Elizabethan times and continued on and off until it closed in 1962. Although the path turns off well before the mine, it passes a small hydro-electric power station (still in use) which, built in 1893 made Greenside mine the first metal mine in the country to have electricity.

From the mine, the walk climbs up towards Lanty's Tarn. Almost at the top, rest on the bench and enjoy the magnificent views of the valley with the fells surrounding it and the lake in the background. Some of the 52 cottages which were built in and around Glenridding to house the miners and their families can be spotted on the other side of the valley.

Lanty's Tarn which was enlarged and dammed in the 1700's by Lancelot (Lanty) Dobson, the owner of Patterdale Hall. He wanted a small lake (tarn) to provide ice all year round. Newly invented Italian ice cream was the fashion and ice was required to keep it cold. When the ice had frozen solid on the tarn, it was cut and kept in an ice house where it remained frozen for 12 months. The mound that housed the ice house can be seen close to the dam.

The walk continues into Grisedale valley and eventually back to Glenridding. If you have time, visit St Patrick's church home to 3 magnificent embroideries worked by Ann Macbeth who trained at the Glasgow school of Art in the early 1900's.

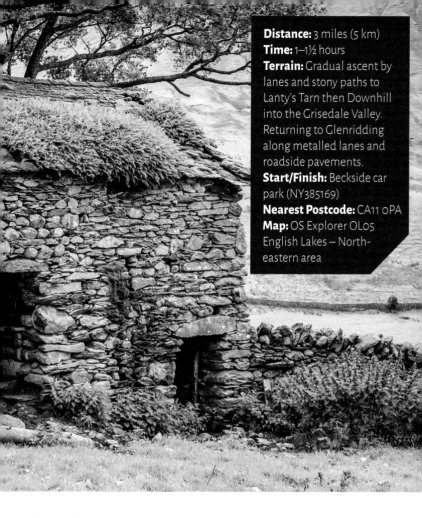

Distance: 3 miles (5 km)
Time: 1–1½ hours
Terrain: Gradual ascent by lanes and stony paths to Lanty's Tarn then Downhill into the Grisedale Valley. Returning to Glenridding along metalled lanes and roadside pavements.
Start/Finish: Beckside car park (NY385169)
Nearest Postcode: CA11 0PA
Map: OS Explorer OL05 English Lakes – North-eastern area

As the walk brings you back into Glenridding look out for the commemoration to Donald Campbell located just past the Steamer pier. In 1955 Campbell broke the water speed record by travelling along Ullswater at 202 miles per hour. Over the next nine years he broke the record six times in the US and in England on the straighter, Coniston Water. It was on Coniston Water in 1967 where a final attempt to go faster cost him his life.

1 Leave the National Park car park past the Information Centre to the A592. Turn right over the bridge then immediately right into a lane past a parade of shops. Continue to a fork in the lane.

2 At the fork bear right slightly downhill to the Glenridding Beck, follow the track past Gillside campsite to a T junction with the lane at Rattlebeck Bridge. Turn left into lane (beware farm traffic) and walk uphill on first a road, then track to a wall corner at Miresbeck House with a sign to Helvellyn.

3 Bear left down to a small wooden bridge across the stream and through a wall into a field. Head diagonally across the field past a waymarker and join a rising stony path skirting woodland above Gillside Farm. Continue along the path gradually gaining height with extensive views of the surrounding fells. Pass through a farm gate set in a wall and then at the next gate turn right up a rising path to a viewpoint with a bench. Enjoy excellent views over the southern reach of Ullswater.

4 Continue downhill and through a gate into Lanty's Tarn. Walk along the path skirting the tarn to the dam wall. Take in the panoramic view of the Grisedale Valley and surrounding fells.

5 Continue downhill on a stony track to a gate in a wall. Turn immediately left through a gate and walk steeply downhill on a grassy path to join a track coming down from the left. Walk down to the bridge over Grisedale Beck. Beyond the bridge at a T junction turn left and follow the minor road until it joins the A592 at Grisedale Bridge.

6 Cross the road (beware traffic) and turn left along the pavement. Join a path on the right skirting the road through trees. At the road again, cross over and turn right along the pavement to join a raised pathway above the road to St.Patrick's boat landing. Recross the road, turn left and follow the pavement back to Glenridding.

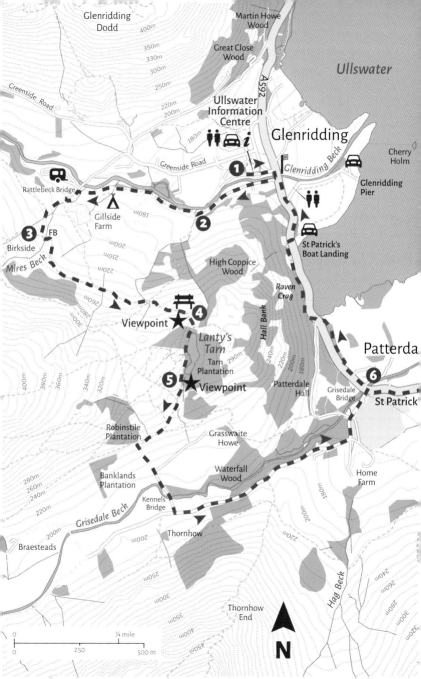

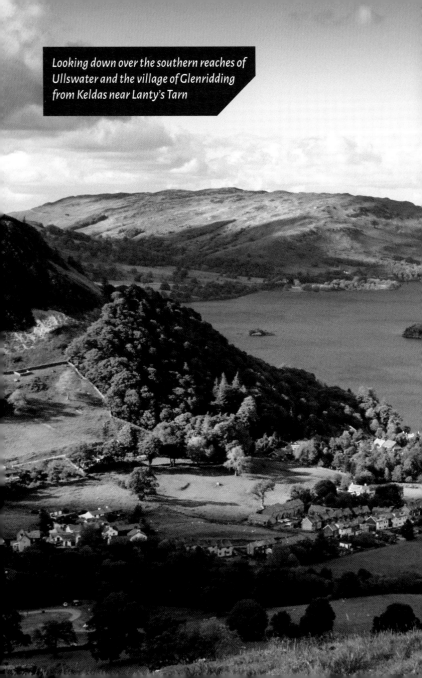
Looking down over the southern reaches of Ullswater and the village of Glenridding from Keldas near Lanty's Tarn

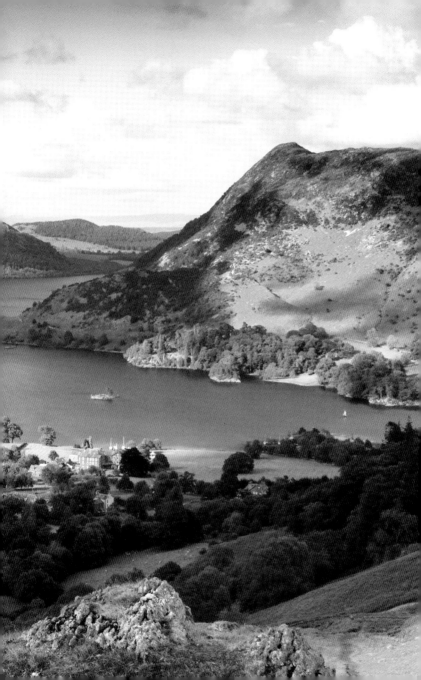

WALK 6
Rosthwaite to Grange

This lovely linear riverside walk in Borrowdale, the largest of the 13 Lakeland valleys, meanders by the clear waters of the river Derwent. Gorgeous autumn hues from the wooded fellsides greets the late season visitor to the area. Borrowdale is home to one of the last surviving fragments of ancient forest in the UK.

The walk starts in the small, pretty village of Rosthwaite, just a short bus-ride from the popular town of Keswick. You'll be walking alongside the serene river Derwent and finishing at the lovely village of Grange, situated at the entrance to the 'Jaws of Borrowdale.'

Grange was owned in medieval times by monks. The name derives from the Latin word granica, meaning granary. The village, as it is now, was developed after the dissolution of the monasteries and the selling of the land to ordinary people. The homes were built of local material with slate roofs mined from nearby.

The double arched packhorse bridge on this walk was built in 1675.

Underneath Castle Crag you'll find the cave of one-time local celebrity Millican Dalton, who spent his summers here living a simple outdoors life, in the first half of the 20th Century.

Nearby Seatoller, is one the wettest inhabited places in England resulting in the verdant lush valley pastures grazed by cattle and the hardy native Herdwick sheep.

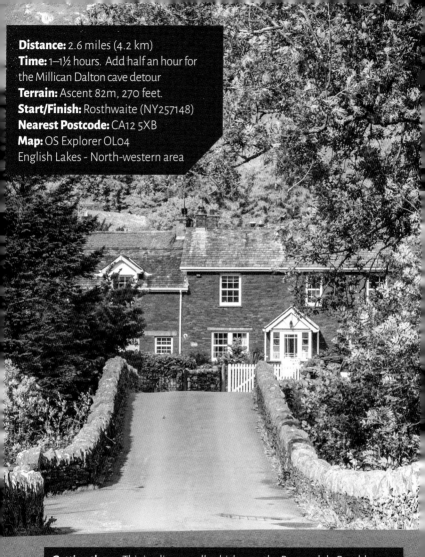

Distance: 2.6 miles (4.2 km)
Time: 1–1½ hours. Add half an hour for the Millican Dalton cave detour
Terrain: Ascent 82m, 270 feet.
Start/Finish: Rosthwaite (NY257148)
Nearest Postcode: CA12 5XB
Map: OS Explorer OL04
English Lakes - North-western area

Getting there: This is a linear walk which uses the Borrowdale Rambler bus. This runs from Keswick to Grange and Rosthwaite throughout the year, with services every half hour in summer, using open top buses for amazing views of the Borrowdale Valley. Hop on the bus in Keswick as there is limited parking in Rosthwaite and no parking in Grange. Operated by Stagecoach, details on Traveline **www.traveline.org.uk**

1 The 78 bus from Keswick stops just before Rosthwaite village. Cross the road, turn right and follow the single road for 150 m to the stone toilet block.

2 Head along the track – the Cumbria Way – which passes a small tearoom on your right.

3 Continue right, past the farm buildings until you reach the stone ford which crosses the River Derwent.

4 Bear right to follow the river on your left and cross over New Bridge, a traditional stone packhorse bridge. Bear right on the main track and pass through a gate.

5 Continue along the riverbank through open fields. Bearing away from the river, continue along the path and pass through a gate into High Hows Wood.

6 Continue through the wood on the Cumbrian Way, passing Castle Crag to the left, where the path goes uphill and becomes rocky, and avoiding minor left paths climb a bank to the highest part of the walk, by a sign-post to Grange and Rosthwaite.

7 Take an optional detour to visit Millican Dalton's cave.

8 Bear right down some rocky steps and through an obvious gap in a dry stone wall. Continue along the rocky steps until you reach the river. Pass through a gate until you reach a junction. You will see another signpost.

9 Turn right and cross a wooden bridge, walking past the campsite on your right.

10 Ignore the track on your left and keep to the right on the road. This will take you directly into Grange.

11 & **12** Turn right into Grange then over a stone bridge to reach the main road (B5289) and bus stop for your return to Keswick.

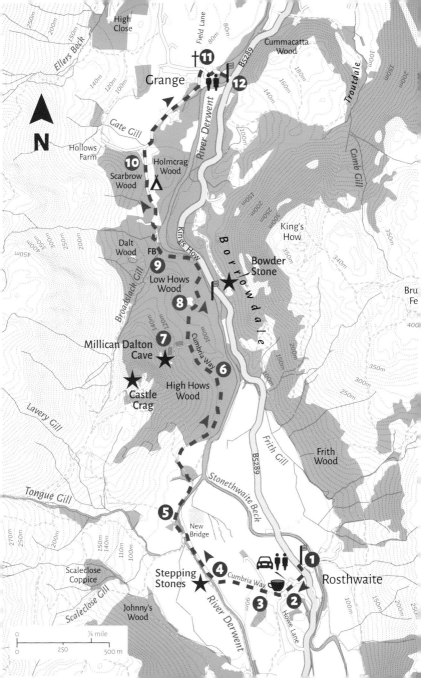

WALK 7
Keswick, Threlkeld and Latrigg

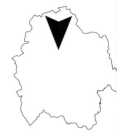

This walk starts from the Tourist Information Centre (TIC) in Keswick, goes along a disused railway to Threlkeld then returns to the start via the summit of Latrigg Fell.

Keswick is situated at the northern end of Derwent Water and is situated between the huge bulk of Skiddaw and the gentle beauty of Derwent Water and the Borrowdale valley. Keswick is the major centre for tourism in the north lakes. This pretty market town offers a wide range of attractions for visitors and is an excellent base for exploring the National Park.

Between Keswick Threlkeld the route follows a section of the 31½-mile Cockermouth Keswick & Penrith Railway which was built between 1862 and 1864, to connect the industrial centres of Workington in the west with Durham in the east via the lofty Stainmore line. It was built primarily with mineral traffic in mind; the first train ran on 26th October 1864. The railway carried passengers from January 1865 to its closure in March 1972. After its closure the four mile section between Keswick and Threlkeld was taken over by the Lake District National Park Authority and converted into a footpath/cycle path

During the flooding caused by Storm Desmond in December 2015 the path was severely damaged, two bridges were completely washed away, one was severely damaged and a section of the route was washed into the river. The path has now been reinstated with two new bridges and the tunnel. It closed when the A66 flyover was constructed, but reopened on Saturday 5 December – the fifth anniversary of Storm Desmond – at a cost approaching £9m.

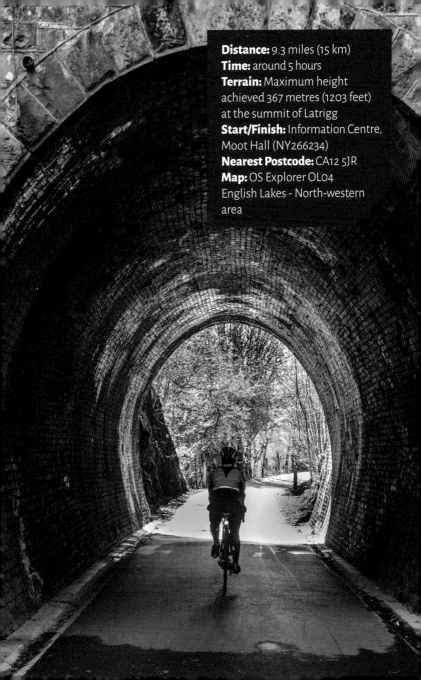

Distance: 9.3 miles (15 km)
Time: around 5 hours
Terrain: Maximum height
achieved 367 metres (1203 feet)
at the summit of Latrigg
Start/Finish: Information Centre,
Moot Hall (NY266234)
Nearest Postcode: CA12 5JR
Map: OS Explorer OL04
English Lakes - North-western
area

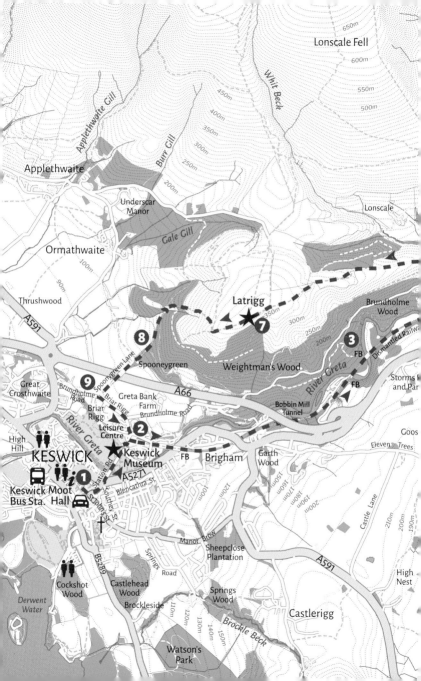

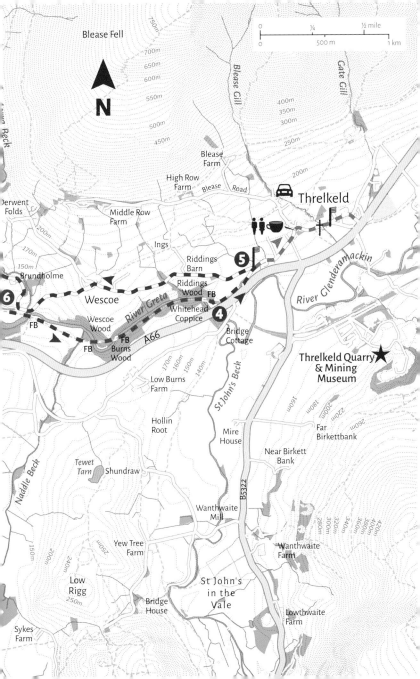

Many walkers will be familiar with the 1932 mass trespass on Kinder Scout in the Peak District. 500 ramblers, protesting against blocked access to areas of countryside, rallied together to highlight the issue.

45 years earlier the Lake District had its own mass trespass on Keswick's iconic Latrigg Fell. At the time, several landowners around Keswick closed footpaths which had been used for generations. A Miss Spedding, then owner of Latrigg, closed the only access paths to the fell and planted a number of trees. In protest, The Keswick Footpath Preservation Association called for a mass trespass. On 1 October 1887, 2,000 people gathered in Keswick and marched to one of the footpaths where they found a chained gate and a "Private" sign. The crowd removed the chains, took down the sign and walked up the footpath singing "Rule Britannia". During a brief court case held at Carlisle a compromise was reached. One footpath, Spooney Green Lane, would be opened to the public while the other would remain private. Following the case, other land owners in the Lake District who had closed footpaths opened them to the public again.

1 From the information Centre in the Moot Hall walk ahead and to your left where you will see the Royal Oak pub. Turn left here and walk along Station Street to the main road. Cross, using the light controlled pedestrian crossing and continue ahead along Station Road, first crossing the bridge over the river Greta, then passing Keswick Museum on your left. Bear slightly left away from the road to pass the Leisure Pool then bear left again. You will soon see the C2C sign at the beginning of the trail you are going to follow, turn right here. After a few yards note the 'Railway Trail 5km' sign on your right. The Railway Trail is open to and very popular with cyclists, walkers, wheelchair users and families so please share the route with care.

2 Carry on until you see a large metal green bridge which you will cross. Just before the bridge a Park Run 2.5 km marker tells enthusiastic runners that they are now halfway along the trail.

3 The trail ends with a short zig zag climb that brings you along the A66 and you follow this for about 100 metres before bearing left onto the approach road to Threlkeld. Soon you will see a narrow road on your left signposted 'Wescoe'. Take this road.

For a low level accessible walk you can turn round here and do the route 'out and back' or catch the hourly bus back to Keswick.

4 Alternative, ignore the 'Wescoe' signpost and walk 200m into Threlkeld which has a coffee shop in the village hall and two pubs.

5 Back on the trail, follow the 'Wescoe' signpost and follow the road to Wescoe with Blencathra rising on your right. As you approach the hamlet take the track that veers off to the left and drops steeply to cross a stone bridge over the Glenderaterra Beck. The track then rises steeply, passing a dwelling on your left. Ignore a footpath sign and also a track on your right. Keep left until you reach a gate, after which you turn right.

6 Pass through the gate and keep to the main track (ignoring a track to your left.) After approximately 800 m you reach a gate across the track. Pass through the gate and bear slightly left, leaving the track to climb up a grassy slope to reach a gate in a stone wall. Beyond the gate the track takes you to the summit of Latrigg.

7 Leaving the summit the track now drops down and you soon meet a Y junction. Keep to the lefthand path and continue down until you meet another track at a T junction where you turn left. The track gets steeper as you descend.

8 Keep to this main path and pass through 2 gates in quick succession. The path then takes you over a bridge which crosses the A66 and you meet a minor road and turn left. This road is narrow and can be busy with traffic so take care and use the footway where possible.

9 Continue to a mini roundabout and bear right to pass the Leisure Centre and Pool where you will join Station Road and can follow your outward route back to the Information Centre in the Moot Hall.

WALK 8
Derwent Water

A richly varied easy walk combines a launch across Derwent Water, a shoreline-hugging path with stunning views and picnic spots, and a wealth of historic, literary and economic points of interest.

The third largest lake in the Lake District by surface area, Derwent Water measures 4.6 km by 1.9 km and is 22 m deep at its deepest. It has 13 islands, is surrounded by forests – some of which are ancient woodlands, and 7 distinct fells.

The Keswick Launch is a scheduled boat service which operates clockwise and anti-clockwise trips around the lake's edge, stopping at 7 different jetties. Each stop offers its own unique interest. For example, High Brandlehow, was the location of a historic lead mine, while Nicol end is a concise sailing marina.

This walk only uses the launch for a single anti-clockwise journey from Keswick to High Brandlehow, but you should explore the other stops if you are staying in the area.

The wood through which the path perambulates is one of the earliest National Trust conservation sites and there are several places of interest to stop along the way. The walk passes a memorial to Thomas Arthur Leonard a 19th-century devotee to walking and outdoor pursuits who founded a holiday club for the less well off, as well as being instrumental in setting up the Youth Hostel Association, the Ramblers Association and the National Trust.

Further along the walk passes Lingholme which is where Beatrix Potter, as a teenager had her family summer holiday

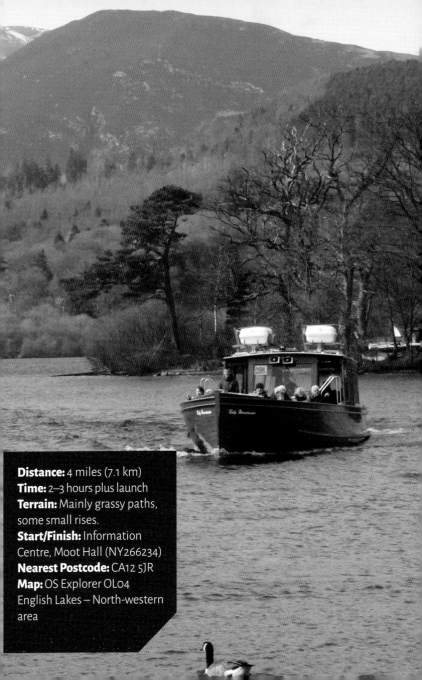

Distance: 4 miles (7.1 km)
Time: 2–3 hours plus launch
Terrain: Mainly grassy paths, some small rises.
Start/Finish: Information Centre, Moot Hall (NY266234)
Nearest Postcode: CA12 5JR
Map: OS Explorer OL04 English Lakes – North-western area

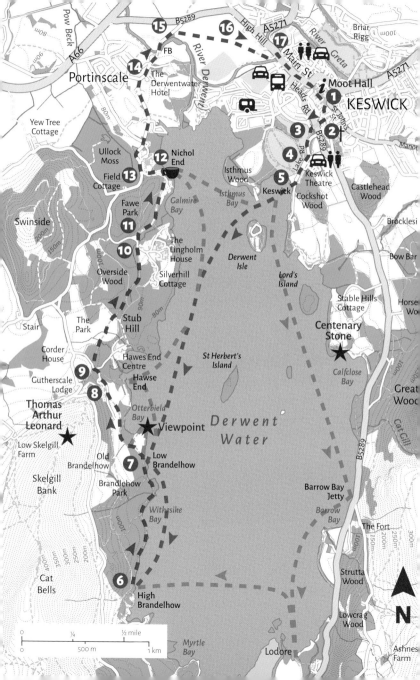

for 10 years commencing in 1890's. It was the landscape around Derwent Water that inspired the early books *The tale of Mrs Tiggle-Winkle* and *The Tale of Squirrel Nutkin*.

Towards the end of the walk just outside Portinscale is a Callendar-Hamilton steel bridge. Originally errected as a temporary replacement for the old stone river Derwent bridge swept away by floods in 1954, it was reconstructed as a pedestrian bridge when the permanent road bridge replacement was finished. It now takes walkers to the fields on which is the annual Keswick Agricultural show.

1 Leave Moot Hall on Lake Road right of the fish & chips takeaway and proceed to the outside of Fisher's.

2 Turn right down a small hill and through the subway.

3 At edge of the park head left and keep the putting green on your right.

4 At car park entrance keep right and continue past Keswick Theatre to Keswick Launch Co. Boat House.

5 Take the Launch to High Brandlehow jetty.

6 Pick up the path on the right through woods and water edge for 1.25 km to Low Brandlehow.

7 Path continues to a headland (worth a visit for the views) but take left path through a gate to Hawes End and Fawe Park.

8 Head on through two gates, passing Hawes End residential Centre, continue into the woods.

9 At a junction of four paths take the second on the right through a narrow gate into woodlands. Path drops down into a clearing before rising, through further woods and reaches Lingholme.

10 Take path diagonally opposite that leads to Fawe Park and Nichol End.

11 Before reaching Fawe Park take right path which descends to Nichol End Marina.

12 Go left to join the access road from Nicol end behind the tea and boat room.

13 When the road is reached turn right and for 800 m continue into Portinscale.

14 As the road bears left there is a large hotel on the right and follow this narrow road past Derwent Outdoor Centre to the metal bridge.

15 After the bridge continue for about 20m where there is a field gate on the right. Go through.

16 Cross the field on a clear path and then against a fence and eventually left to meet the B5289.

17 Turn right and follow the road to traffic lights. Head straight over into a pedestrian area and to Moot Hall (500 m in total).

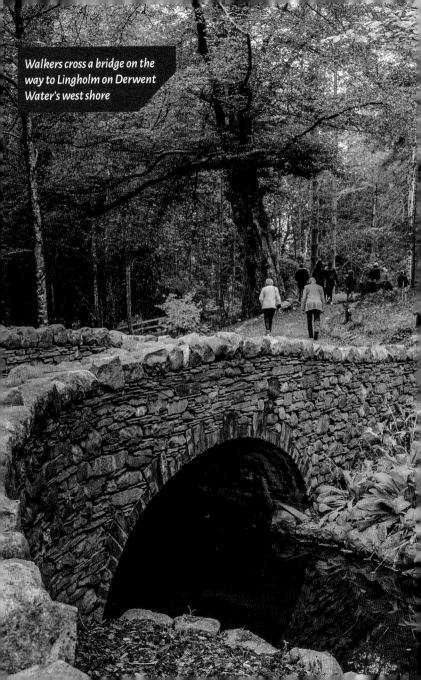

Walkers cross a bridge on the way to Lingholm on Derwent Water's west shore

WALK 9
Buttermere

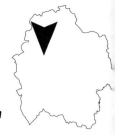

A delightful walk, popular from the Victorian times, with stunning views and picnic spots.

This walk – a favourite of many Lake District visitors – is a smashing little walk for all the family. It is mainly along the lake side and on a nice day, offers splendid views throughout. There is even a little section through a tunnel for the kids to enjoy.

The walk encircles Buttermere Lake – the first of three adjacent valley lakes that is 1.25 km long, 0.25 km wide and 23 m deep. The lake is set in a crag enclosed tree-clad bowl, which temporarily cuts the walker off from the rest of civilisation. Both the village and the lake derive their names from the 10th Century Norseman chief "Buther" and "mere" meaning lake. On a sunny day the lake water is unaccountable green and shimmery but in winter the whole area can feel remote, wild and windy.

Buttermere village has several sights worth investigating. St James is a small church built entirely from stones taken from the bed of Sourmilk Gill – a narrow but fast stream cascading from Red Pike. There is also the former "Fish Inn" now Buttermere Court, a hotel which was the home of Mary Robinson the "Maid of Buttermere" who was decieved into a bigamous marriage in 1802 to John Hatfield – an impersonator and forger who was eventually hung in Carlisle. The Maid of Buttermere is mentioned in William Wordsworth's *The Prelude* and is the subject of a novel of that name by Melvyn Bragg.

To the north of the village, between Buttermere and Crummock Water, Rannerdale Knotts is known for its spring Bluebell carpet.

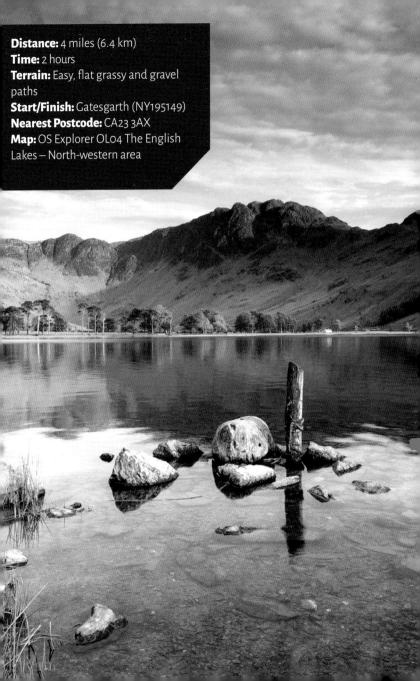

Distance: 4 miles (6.4 km)
Time: 2 hours
Terrain: Easy, flat grassy and gravel paths
Start/Finish: Gatesgarth (NY195149)
Nearest Postcode: CA23 3AX
Map: OS Explorer OL04 The English Lakes – North-western area

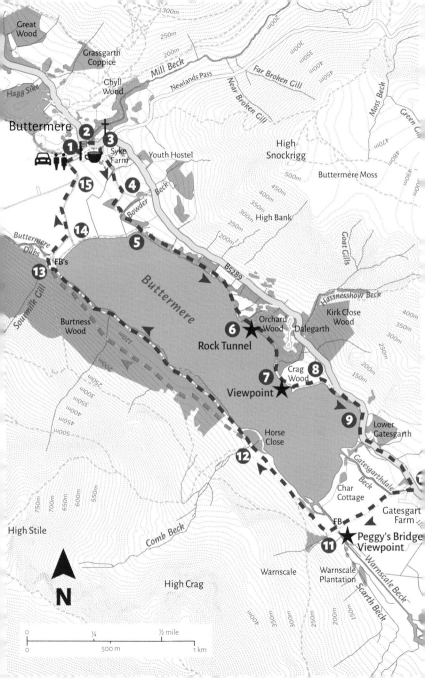

1 Start from outside Buttermere Court, the Lake District car park (with WC's) and the bus stop. Alternatively you may want to start from the car park at point 10 – that way if you are walking at a slower pace, you can break your walk in Buttermere village where there are pubs providing refreshments.

2 Retrace to the junction of the main road B5289 and turn right up a hill, until a broad opening/gate on the right (3) leads to a Tearoom and Syke farm.

3 Go through the farm and onto the open fields as the Lake comes into view.

4 Head right through a gate and down a rocky bank to join the lakeshore path.

5 Keeping the lake on your right continue through the open woods, several gates and over a stream bridge until a rock tunnel hewn out for a Manchester Mill owner is reached.

6 Tall walkers will bend their heads, a phone torch will help in the initial steps and children will love the echoes. After crossing a bridge, swing around right to Shingle Point for a classic viewpoint.

7 Continue on the broad path adjacent to the lake as it rises.

8 Divert right on the narrower lake shore path which after a short time meets the main road.

9 Follow the road (be careful as there is no path), for 500 m until, going over a small stone bridge Gatesgarth farm is reached.

10 Immediately after the bridge turn right, through a gate and onto a single track with Gatesgarthdale Beck on the right and the farm on your left. Stay on the track until you reach a gate onto the lake plain. Cross Peggy's Bridge and turn right after next gate.

11 The path, now on open fell with a wall above the lake on the right continues 700 m before Comb Beck is reached. The beck drains the highest of the Trio fells of High Stile and is marked by a plaque seat.

12 Cross a bridge and then just after the path divides. Either continue along the lake side path or take a grassy track on the left, leading up the hill to walk through Burtness Wood. After 1.6 km the paths meet at a junction prior to Sourmilk Gill.

13 Take the right path through a gate and go over one bridge and then immediately over a second bridge and follow the path round the foot of the lake.

14 Leaving the lake path go left through a gate.

15 Follow the wide track to reach Buttermere Court.

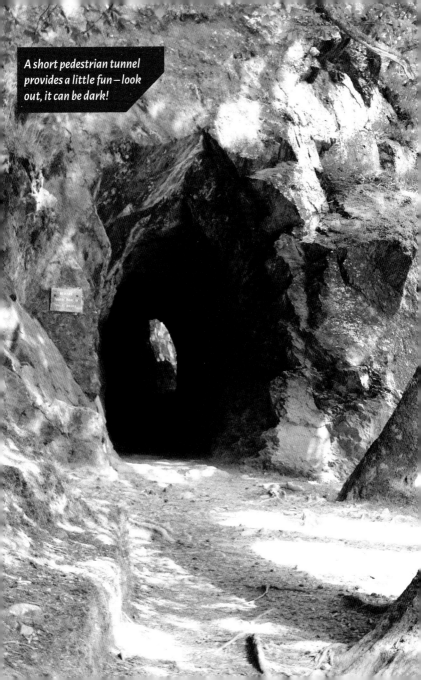

A short pedestrian tunnel provides a little fun — look out, it can be dark!

WALK 10
Friars Crag

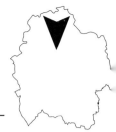

*Part of the 'loveliest square mile in Lakeland' –
Alfred Wainwright (Lakeland walk's author)*

A short and leisurely walk (1.3 km or 0.8 of a mile) from the
Information Centre in the Moot Hall Keswick to Friars Crag,
with outstanding views and interest. From the viepoint at Friars
Crag, at the bottom of Derwent Water, there is a clear view
south to the 'Jaws of Borrowdale'. In the distance is the Scafell
Range, the highest in England.

The walk starts in Keswick. Many people think Keswick gets its
name from an Old English version of "Cheese Market" with the
town getting its market charter in 1276 and still having a market
to this day on Thursdays and Saturdays.

It's a pretty simple walk from the town centre to Friars Crag
taking you to the lake shore and then following it to the south.
The path is suitable for all. Just before the crag is a memorial to
John Ruskin, the 19th century writer, thinker, and painter.
Ruskin's first memory was being taken to Friar's Crag. He was
an inspiration to the National Trust founders, and the
foundation is encapsulated on a plaque to the left as you approach the viewpoint from the town.

Derwent Water has four major islands all owned by National
Trust. The first is Derwent Isle (passed on the way to the viewpoint) with its private residence. It is open to the public just 5
days annually. Once at the viewpoint, looking down the middle
of the lake you can see St Herbert's Island used as a hermit-
age. St Herbert brought Christianity to the area in 685AD and

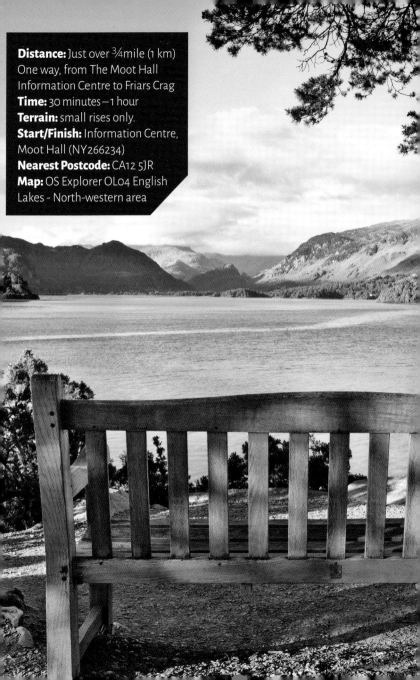

Distance: Just over ¾mile (1 km)
One way, from The Moot Hall
Information Centre to Friars Crag
Time: 30 minutes – 1 hour
Terrain: small rises only.
Start/Finish: Information Centre,
Moot Hall (NY266234)
Nearest Postcode: CA12 5JR
Map: OS Explorer OL04 English
Lakes - North-western area

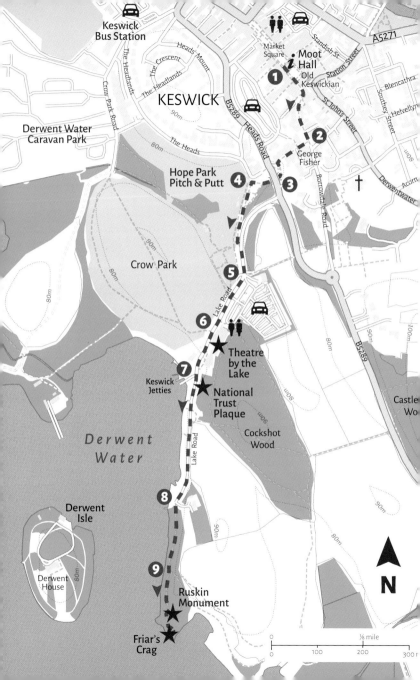

Keswick
Bus Station

Derwent Water
Caravan Park

The Crescent

The Headlands

The Headlands

Heads Mount

Crow Park Road

The Headlands

KESWICK

90m

80m

The Heads

Market
Square

Standish St

Station Street

A5271

Moot
Hall

Old
Keswickian

St John's Street

Blencathra

Southey Street

Helvellyn

Derwent Acorn

1

2

George Fisher

3

Borrowdale Road

Derwentwater

Hope Park
Pitch & Putt

4

Crow Park

90m

80m

80m

5

Lake Road

6

Theatre by the
Lake

7

Keswick
Jetties

National
Trust
Plaque

Cockshot
Wood

Castle
Wo

80m

90m

100m

D e r w e n t
W a t e r

Lake Road

8

Derwent Isle

Derwent
House

80m

90m

9

Ruskin
Monument

Friar's
Crag

90m

80m

B5289

B5289 Heads Road

Heads Road

N

0   ⅛ mile

0   100   200   300 m

was visited by Friars who departed from "Friars Crag". On the left is Lord's Island, past home of the Earls of Derwentwater, and the ruin of a manor house. Nowadays, Lord's Island and lastly the small Rampsholme Island beyond, are both wildlife refuges.

Still at the viewpoint – to your right (west, across the lake), are the high fells of Cat Bells and Maiden Moor. To the left is Walla Crag. Directly opposite is Lingholm where a young Beatrix Potter holidayed in summer.

1 Leave The Information Centre at the Moot Hall and walk to the right of The Old Keswickian fish & chips take-away. Proceed to the outside of George Fisher's.

2 Turn right down a small hill to the bottom of the road.

3 Go through the subway on the left.

4 At edge of the park turn left and keep the putting green on your right. The small park with its collection of benches, is a lovely spot to rest, admire the flowers and hopefully see a few birds – robins and blackbirds are common here.

5 At car park entrance keep right and up small rise to WC's on left and then pass the Theatre on the Lake.

6 Pass Crow Park Entrance on the right with HRH Prince Charles plaque. Proceed downhill to the Keswick Launch jetties – try not to get pecked by the duck and geese who congregate here to be fed by tourists.

7 Turn to the left on lake promenade passing National Trust plaque.

8 At Crossing of paths stay by edge of the lake.

9 Path divides for Shandshag Bay and Ruskin Monument. Keep right on path to Friars Crag. Return by the same route.

WALK 11
Tarn Hows, Lake and Trees

An easy walk through a Victorian Estate where natural beauty and human artifice have been harmoniously combined. The route passes some typical Cumbrian farmhouses with literary associations and starts at the head of lovely Coniston water.

From Monk Coniston the route passes Low Yewdale Farm where Arthur Ransome spent his summer holidays as a young man, later using it as his model for Dixon's Farm in Swallows and Amazons. It later passes Yew Tree Farm with its traditional Spinning Gallery. This stood in for "Hill Top", Beatrix Potter's farm in the 2006 film, "Miss Potter".

From Tom Gill car park the route climbs Tom Gill passing delightful waterfalls resplendent in dappled sunshine – weather permitting. It emerges at Tarn Hows, part of the Monk Coniston estate, originally owned by the monks of Furness Abbey. Later wealthy Victorian owners created an arboretum around the house and perhaps more significantly dammed the outlet of three small tarns in the upper part of the estate to create the Tarn Hows that is seen today. The tarn is one of the district's most famed beauty spots with lovely views of the distant fells.

Descending from the tarn an arboretum is encountered. Along the Tree Trail there are over 50 species of tree and shrub from all over the world. Spring showcases the azaleas and rhododendrons, while autumn the red of the Japanese Maples. After passing through the walled garden and visiting the gazebo it is a short stroll back to Coniston Water.

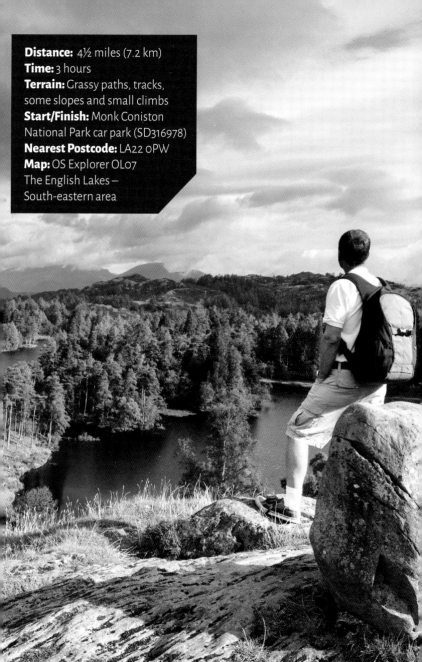

Distance: 4½ miles (7.2 km)
Time: 3 hours
Terrain: Grassy paths, tracks, some slopes and small climbs
Start/Finish: Monk Coniston National Park car park (SD316978)
Nearest Postcode: LA22 0PW
Map: OS Explorer OL07 The English Lakes – South-eastern area

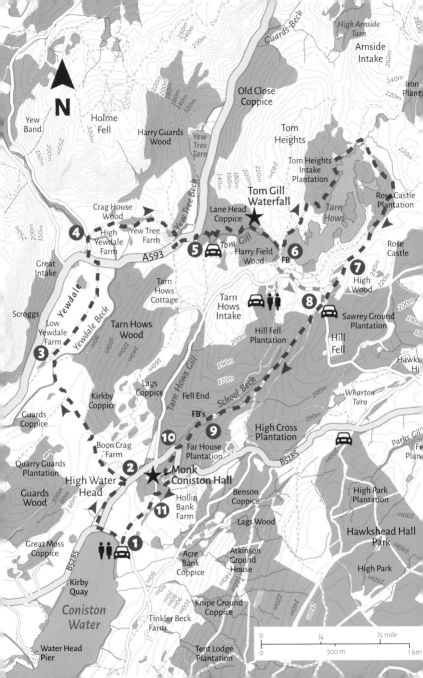

1 The walk starts at Monk Coniston National Park car park. Leave the car park, cross the minor road, turn left to follow the roadside path to meet the Coniston-Hawkshead road (B5285). Cross the road and turn right along the roadside path to Boon Crag farm.

2 Turn left signed Low Yewdale. Pass through the farm buildings, and follow the bridleway for 850 m before crossing a bridge and bearing right to Low Yewdale farm.

3 Follow path signed High Yewdale across 4 fields to reach the A593 at High Yewdale. Cross the road, turn left and then right after 60 m onto a minor road (signed Hodge Close), to Shepherd's Bridge.

4 Cross the bridge and turn right and follow bridleway to reach Yew Tree farm. Cross the A593 diagonally right to a wicket gate and once through the gate turn sharp left and follow a permissive path, parallel to the road. Cross a footbridge and pass through a parking area, to reach Tom Gill (aka Glen Mary) National Trust car park.

5 From the NT noticeboard, cross the bridge, and take the footpath signed Tarn Hows, through the woods (do not cross the beck and at a path junction just before the main falls, keep right) to ascend Tom Gill, keeping the Gill to your right, and arriving after about 650 m, at Tarn Hows.

6 You are now at a junction in the paths.

Optional: At this point the main walk heads off on a circuit around the Tarn. This circuit can be omitted which will shorten the walk by 2.6 km or 1.7 miles. To omit the circuit turn right at this point and climb up the track leading away from the Tarn to reach the tarmac minor access road. Turn left and walk along the road for about 400 m to reach the car park at Point 8.

To continue with the main walk route around the Tarn, turn left and follow the path by the water's edge. This path continues in an obvious route around the Tarn, staying close to the water all of the way round.

7 At a path junction on far side of the Tarn (about ¾ of the way round), turn half left (signed Hawkshead) to join an elevated path and continue on to reach a gate into a car park.

8 Across the road opposite the entrance to the car park, pass through wooden field gate, to follow the path downhill through Hill Fell Plantation (do not take path to Hawkshead on left.) After a short distance bear right at a junction and follow path signed Coniston and Boon Crag. Descend for 1 km or so following signs to Coniston until a left turn signed Monk Coniston.

9 Follow this path which crosses a narrow footbridge across a dam crest, and continue to the B5285.

10 Cross the road to enter Monk Coniston Hall grounds and explore the Tree Trail signs. Continue through the walled garden and visit the Gazebo.

11 Exit the estate and proceed south west across a grassy pasture to reach the minor road and return to the car park.

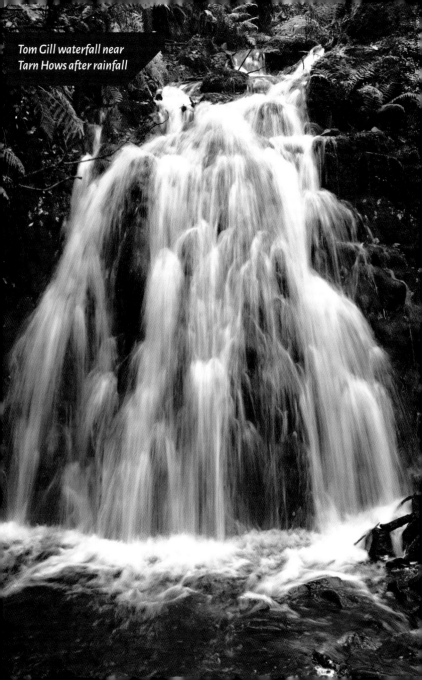

Tom Gill waterfall near Tarn Hows after rainfall

WALK 12
Coniston Copper Trail

This is a walk to discover the mining history and archaeology of a beautiful valley under the soaring crags of the Coniston mountain range.

The Coppermines Valley lies directly behind Coniston village between the long high ridge of the main Coniston Fells and the outlying summit of Wetherlam. This impressively steep valley has been of great interest to miners from as far back as Elizabethan times and this walk will guide you round some of the main sites. There are interpretative notices on the route.

You can visit remains of engine houses and waterwheels dating from between 1595 and 1900. Old workings and mines can be dangerous and should not be entered.

Looking down on to the valley floor from the elevated walk, the remains of a vast copper processing factory with heaps of waste slag can be seen. As you take in the stunning views, imagine what this peaceful valley was like at its industrial peak in the 1800's with the noise of many workers and machinery and the rush of the powerful water wheels.

The highest point of the walk is beautiful Levers Water which is a naturally occurring tarn dammed to supply water to the mines and the village. Footpaths here lead up to the high fells.

The Ruskin Museum, near the start of the walk in the village, has displays and information about the history of the village. There has also been an interesting conservation project: Coniston Copper **https://www.lakedistrict.gov.uk/learning/ archaeologyhistory/coniston-copper**

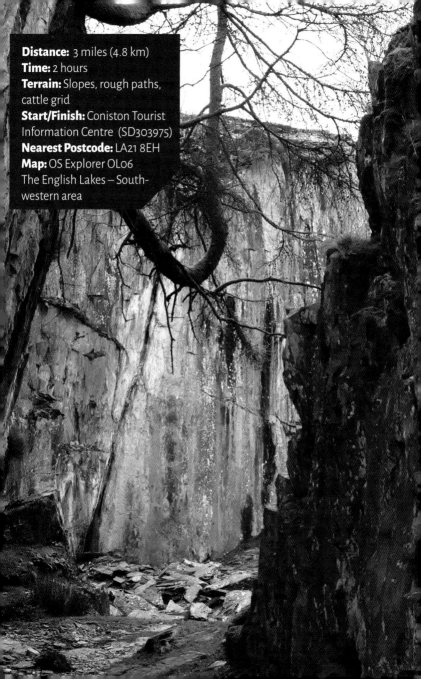

Distance: 3 miles (4.8 km)
Time: 2 hours
Terrain: Slopes, rough paths, cattle grid
Start/Finish: Coniston Tourist Information Centre (SD303975)
Nearest Postcode: LA21 8EH
Map: OS Explorer OL06 The English Lakes – South-western area

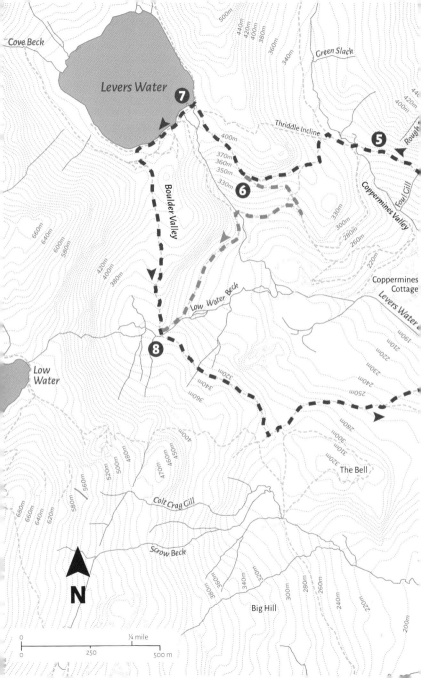

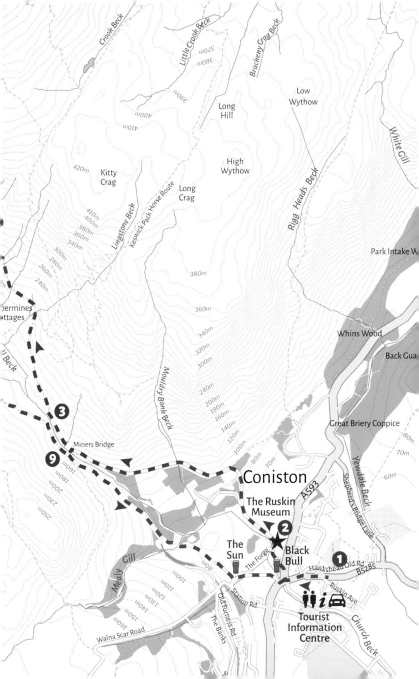

1 Turn left out of the carpark and then bear left. At the main road (A 593) turn right. Cross the road and take the lane between the Black Bull pub and the village store.

2 Follow the road past the museum and up the hill to where it becomes the track to Coniston Copper Mines. Continue over a cattle grid and past Miners Bridge on the left.

3 Opposite the hydroelectric scheme take a track to the right. Further up the hill, ignore the path on the left leading to the row of historical Irish Miners Cottages. Turn left at the footpath junction and continue along the path above the valley.

4 Pass a glaciated rock on the right with the name J Mara inscribed with the date 1887. As the track rises, the ore dressing floor and relocated waterwheel can be seen below. The Old Engine workings can be seen in the distance further along the path. The mine shaft, to the right just before the buildings, may be entered up to the security fence (torch required).

5 Continue along the track to cross a bridge to visit the New Engine workings and wheel pit with its dramatic story.

6 Bear left keeping the wheel pit on your right and walk up hill on a faint track to reach a water leat. Walk along the banking, passing under Kernal Crag to reach a rough track and turn right. Proceed steeply uphill to Levers Water.

7 Cross the dam via the spillway weir and continue along the side of the water. At the end of the dam, keep left to join a rising path towards a wire fence to observe the entrance to Back Strings copper mine. Continue along a path, following the fence, which turns left up hill. Stay on the path initially up hill, then descending down Boulder Valley. Cross a footbridge to reach Pudding Stone (a very large single boulder).

Alternative route - if it is not possible to cross the dam, retrace the route down the stony track. Turn right at the first path junction after about 0.5 km and follow a footpath up to Pudding Stone (see 7).

8 Continue along the footpath to reach a junction of footpaths at Crowberry Haws. Turn left and immediately left again downhill and back to Miners Bridge.

9 Do not cross the bridge, continue down the track. On meeting the road turn left to pass the Sun Inn and down into the village.

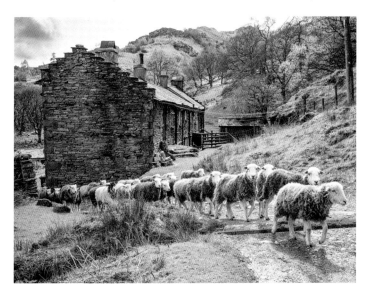

WALK 13
Eskdale and Stanley Ghyll

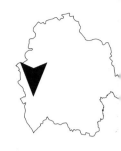

Relax in the beautiful Eskdale valley where industrial heritage is never far away.

The River Esk starts life up on the Scafell massif before meandering its way through the glaciated Eskdale valley where the river forms a series of tranquil pools and lively cascades. This short circular walks starts at the terminus of the Ravenglass and Eskdale Railway, La'al Ratty, at Dalegarth – originally built to service the local iron ore mines. The walk to Gill Force covers a delightful stretch of the River Esk and Girder Bridge is a reminder of the iron ore mining heritage. If the river is low Gill Force is a great place to bask on the rocks and maybe dip your toes in the water.

Take time out to visit the diminutive and stunningly located 12th century church of St. Catherine. The nearby stepping stones across the river also provide an interesting diversion when the water is low.

The approach to Dalegarth Falls (Stanley Falls) passes through some delightful mixed woodland before entering the dramatic deep and narrow Stanley Ghyll gorge. The habitat here is distinctly "Jurassic" in character with ferns, mosses, lichens, exotic feeling rhododendrons and numerous small waterfalls. Plunging 20 m (60 ft) into a dark pool Dalegarth Force (Stanley Force) is surely one of the loveliest in the Lakes.

The walks starts from Dalegarth Station which is reached by car or "La'al Ratty" steam train from Ravenglass.

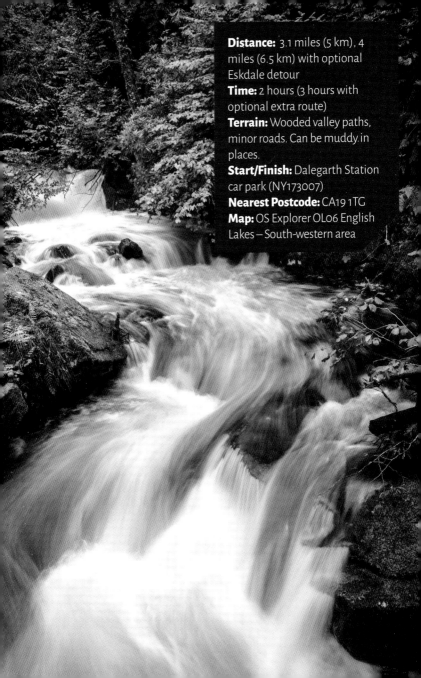

Distance: 3.1 miles (5 km), 4 miles (6.5 km) with optional Eskdale detour
Time: 2 hours (3 hours with optional extra route)
Terrain: Wooded valley paths, minor roads. Can be muddy in places.
Start/Finish: Dalegarth Station car park (NY173007)
Nearest Postcode: CA19 1TG
Map: OS Explorer OL06 English Lakes – South-western area

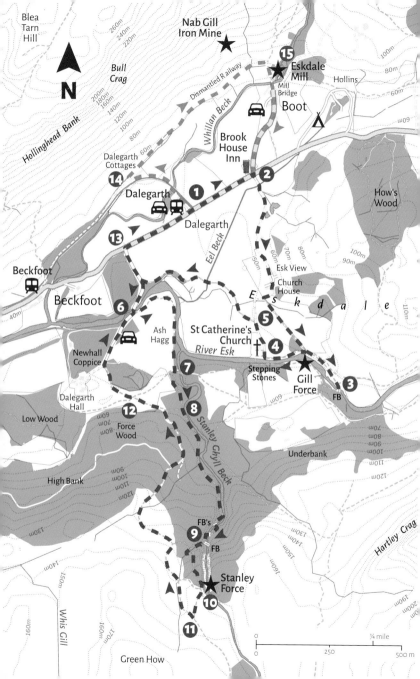

1 Leave the station and turn left onto the valley road and follow the road to the Brook House Inn.

2 Turn right, signed St Catherine's Church 600 yds, and follow the lane south past Esk View Farm bearing right past Church House and then in about 40m turn left through a wicket gate signed Gill Force, Girder Bridge 400 yds. Follow the old mineral railway in a south east direction, having passed through a field gate/wicket gate combination, to reach Gill Force and the "Girder Bridge".

3 After viewing the Falls (cascade) just after the bridge, return along the same path but bear left at the first junction and follow the riverside path to reach St Catherine's church.

4 Leave the church by the metal gate, turn left and then, after 100 m turn left to join Parsons Passage, signed Dalegarth Station 800 yds.

5 Follow the path until you reach a minor road. Turn left onto the road.

6 Cross the river bridge and immediately turn left (Anne's Walk). Follow the path signed Dalegarth Falls 900 yards, through two sets of gates and along the riverside.

7 Pass through wicket gate at end of Anne's Walk and at next path junction go ahead, signed Dalegarth Falls ¼ mile, along path which follows a wall (keep wall on right hand side). Where wall turns right stay on the path (away from the wall corner) and continue for another 50 m, to a junction with a footpath coming in from right.

8 Join this clearly signed path to the Falls which heads off beside the beck. After almost 700 m cross a wooden footbridge and follow the path on the east side of the gorge before reaching a second footbridge which takes you back across to the west side of the gorge. Continue following the path until you come to a third footbridge

9 **Do not cross this bridge** but turn sharp right to ascend a stone path with a wooden handrail. At the top of this short ascent bear left and, after crossing a small stone slab bridge, keep left to climb the access path to the viewing platform.

Eskdale and Stanley Ghyll | Lake District 83

10 Leave the Falls and follow the path upwards for about 60 m and pass through a field gate and walk forwards until your path comes up to a bridleway.

11 Turn right onto the bridleway and follow it downhill through two field gates (always keeping left if your path meets another from the right) until you meet a four way path junction at the bottom of the slope.

12 Follow path ahead (north west) signed Dalegarth Station 850 yds, pass through a field gate and follow the minor road, past Trough House Bridge car park. Continue on the minor road past the entrance to Anne's Walk (which you took on your outbound route at point 6.) Stay on the road and follow it as it bends to the left until it joins with the main road.

13 Turn right and head up the road for 270 m to reach the station.

Optional: Continue the walk to visit Eskdale Mill – an additional circular distance of 1.45 km (0.9 miles). From the station walk to the end of the platform. **Check that departure/arrival of trains is not imminent!** When you are sure it is safe and no trains are due, descend onto the railway, cross the bridge then keep to the right of the tracks to reach the end of a terrace of cottages.

14 Turn sharp right passing behind the cottages, to join a grassy footpath, along an old railway track, for about 600 m to a bridleway junction and turn right, passing through a field gate, to reach Eskdale Mill.

15 Once you have had a look around follow the village street south to reach the Brook House Inn (point 2 of the original walk), where you turn right to return to Dalegarth Station.

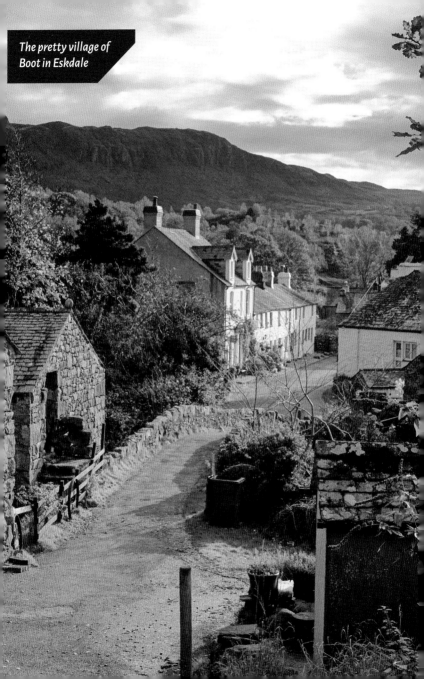

The pretty village of
Boot in Eskdale

WALK 14
Silver How

This delightful fell overlooks the village of Grasmere in the central Lake District. Despite being less than half the height of the highest Lakeland fell, the views from the summit in all directions are extensive.

From the top of Silver How you will see a number of the principal Lakeland fells including Blencathra, Helvellyn, Fairfield, Crinkle Crags, Bowfell and the Landale Pikes and of course Helm Crag with its famous "Lion and Lamb" rocks at the summit. Silver How overlooks Grasmere tarn. Other sections of visible water include Rydal Water, Loughrigg Tarn, the upper reaches of Windermere and a small section of Coniston Water.

Grasmere itself was the home of the best known of the lake poets – William Wordsworth who with his sister Dorothy moved into Dove Cottage in 1799 and they stayed here until 1808 when they moved to Allan Bank. For more on Wordsworth, see walk 16, (page 96). Allan Bank – now a National Trust property – is open to the public. It was also the home of Hardwicke Rawnsley who is remembered chiefly for his preservation work in the Lake District and as a founder of the National Trust.

Grasmere is also famous for Grasmere Gingerbread. It was invented in 1854 by Victorian cook Sarah Nelson in the village from where it gets its name. A unique, spicy-sweet cross between a biscuit and cake, try some!

The walk is graded as moderate and follows public footpaths and well-trodden paths over the open fells.

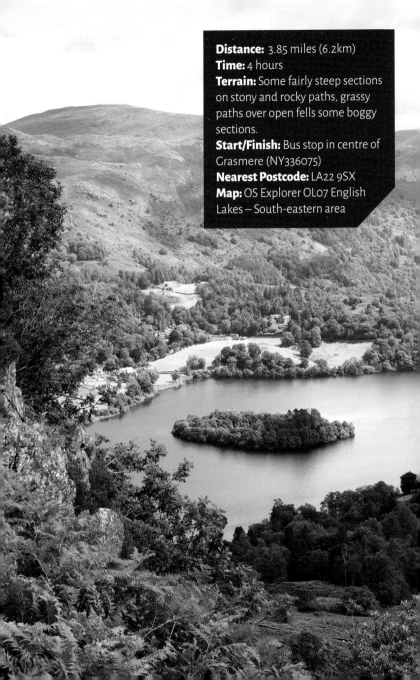

Distance: 3.85 miles (6.2km)
Time: 4 hours
Terrain: Some fairly steep sections on stony and rocky paths, grassy paths over open fells some boggy sections.
Start/Finish: Bus stop in centre of Grasmere (NY336075)
Nearest Postcode: LA22 9SX
Map: OS Explorer OL07 English Lakes – South-eastern area

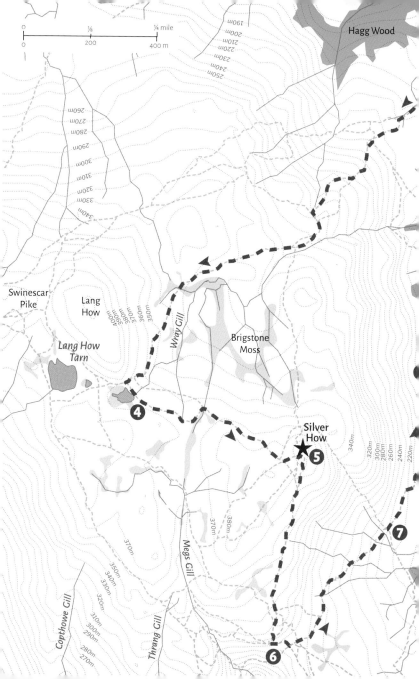

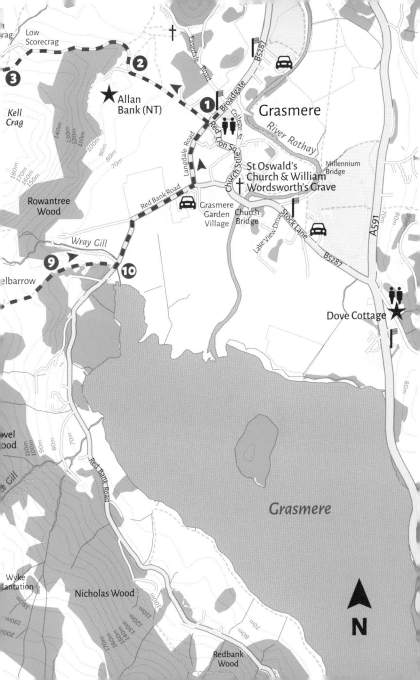

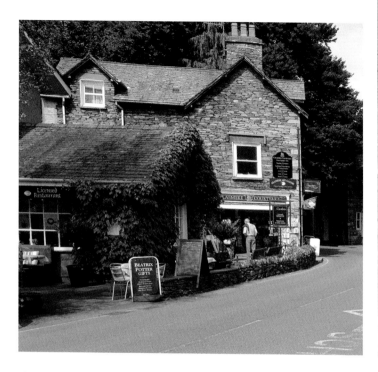

1 From the bus stop(s) in Broadgate walk south west along Broadgate. Where Broadgate meets Langdale road turn right up a narrow tarmacadam road. There is a National Trust sign pointing to Allan Bank on the wall. Where the road passes through two stone pillars you can bypass the cattle grid by going through a small gateway on the left. Ignore the first footpath on right, pass through an avenue of trees and before arriving at Allan Bank take the second footpath on the right with a small National Trust signpost – Path to Silver How. This is initially a tarmacadam path.

2 Continue along this rising path to arrive at a property on your right. Bear left here signposted Silver How & Langdale. The path becomes much rougher underfoot with loose stones and rocks. Pass through two kissing gates and just beyond the second at a wall corner keep ahead on the path which ascends a grassy slope.

❸ The path continues upwards passing through a stand of juniper. There is a fairly steep drop on your right into a gill. Keep right at a path junction and follow the path for approximately half a mile (800 metres) over open country in a south westerly direction to meet a crossing path near a small tarn on your left, turn left along this path. This last section of path may be very feint in places and may also be boggy in places.

❹ Continue along this well-defined path to the summit of Silver How with its stone cairn and spectacular views.

❺ From the summit descend in a southerly direction on a fairly well defined track to reach a large stone cairn. Just before the cairn bear right on a descending path to meet a crossing path. Turn left along this new path.

❻ Soon arrive at crossing of paths at a stone cairn. Turn left and continue ahead, ignoring paths to the left and right, in a north easterly direction until you meet a dry stone wall. Please note that there are three fairly awkward beck crossings along this path.

❼ At the wall bear left (north east) to follow the descending path alongside the wall. This next section of path is fairly stony and rocky.

❽ Pass through two kissing gates then a third gate after which the path passes through woodland between dry stone walls

❾ The path passes through a fourth gate to meet Red Bank Road.

❿ Turn left along Red Bank Road and just before the garden centre turn left along Langdale road to arrive back at the bus stop(s).

WALK 15
Wasdale Wonder

Explore lovely Wasdale – one of the quieter parts of the district but one of the most beautiful.

The walk follows the banks of the River Irt, crossing over it at Lund Bridge – a typical Cumbrian packhorse bridge. On emerging by the side of Wast Water – the deepest lake in England – there are views of Wasdale screes as they plunge from nearly 2000 feet ending unseen 250 feet beneath the surface of the lake.

Looking up the lake the famous ring of fells can be seen – Yewbarrow, Kirkfell, Great Gable and the Scafells – the view featured by the Lake District National Park in their logo.

Near the lake shore is Wasdale Hall, built by a wealthy banker, and now a Youth Hostel. Leaving the lake, the route returns along footpaths through mature woodland, open country and passes farmhouses and fields.

The walk starts near Nether Wasdale, a charming village, with a 16th century church, village green, Victorian maypole and 2 pubs.

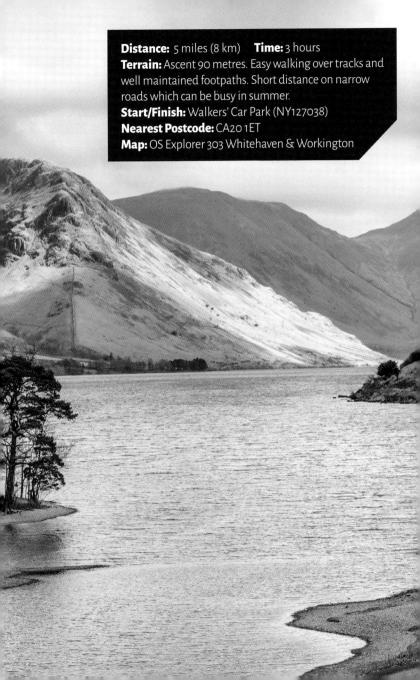

Distance: 5 miles (8 km)　　**Time:** 3 hours
Terrain: Ascent 90 metres. Easy walking over tracks and well maintained footpaths. Short distance on narrow roads which can be busy in summer.
Start/Finish: Walkers' Car Park (NY127038)
Nearest Postcode: CA20 1ET
Map: OS Explorer 303 Whitehaven & Workington

1 Turn right out the carpark, cross Forest Bridge and turn left on to a public footpath signposted Wast Water. Follow this track to Easthwaite Farm. Just before the farm go through a gate on the left, sign posted Wasdale Head, bypassing the farm. Bear left after passing through a gate to rejoin the track. Continue ahead until just before the second gate across the track.

2 Just before the second field gate, turn left through a kissing gate into the woods. Keep along the riverbank downstream to the packhorse bridge. Cross the bridge, go through another kissing gate, on the right, into Low Wood. Follow the path, keeping right, down to the river again and continue upstream to the lakeshore. Walk along the lake shore, passing Wasdale Hall, to join the road and turn right.

3 Turn left at the first road junction, following a road sign to Gosforth.

4 After Greendale and immediately after a bridge over the beck turn left off the road, through a gate onto a wooded path by the beck signposted Galesyke. Continue along the path, turn right at the wall and pass through the gate.

5 Continue ahead through more open country along a grassy path, passing a rocky outcrop on the left. Pass through a gate and keep straight ahead following way marks (yellow dots) through 2 more gates.

6 After passing through the second gate, turn sharp right, signposted to Scale Bridge. After 100 metres, pass through the right hand gate and keep ahead to a T junction of paths. Turn left, signposted to Mill Place. Continue ahead following a bridleway sign to Cinderdale Bridge. Go through the farmyard to reach the road. Turn right, then immediately left to follow the road back to the car park.

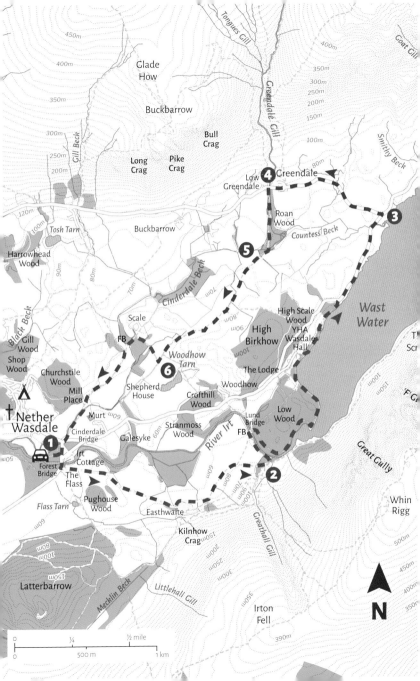

450m

400m

350m

Glade
How

Tongues Gill

Coat Gill

Buckbarrow

400m

350m

300m

250m

200m

150m

100m

Greendale Gill

Bull
Crag

300m

Gill Beck

Long
Crag

Pike
Crag

250m

200m

80m

Low
Greendale

4 Greendale

Smithy Beck

100m

120m

Tosh Tarn

100m

Buckbarrow

90m

Roan
Wood

Countess Beck

3

Harrowhead
Wood

80m

Cinderdale Beck

5

70m

Wast
Water

Black Beck

Scale

80m

70m

High Scale
Wood

Gill
Wood

FB

90m

Woodhow
Tarn

6

High
Birkhow

YHA
Wasdale
Hall

T
Scr

Shop
Wood

Churchstile
Wood

The Lodge

100m

Mill
Place

Shepherd
House

Woodhow

'F' G

Murt

60m

Crofthill
Wood

Nether
Wasdale

Cinderdale
Bridge

Stranmoss
Wood

River Irt

Lund
Bridge

Low
Wood

Great Gully

1

Galesyke

60m

FB

150m

50m

Forest
Bridge

Irt
Cottage

2

The
Flass

80m

70m

Cre>thall Gill

Whin
Rigg

Flass Tarn

Pughouse
Wood

Easthwaite

100m

60m

Kilnhow
Crag

150m

Irton
Fell

500m

Latterbarrow

80m

100m

150m

Mecklin Beck

Littlehall Gill

200m

250m

300m

350m

390m

450m

400m

N

0   ¼   ½ mile

0   500 m   1 km

WALK 16
Grasmere and Rydal

Wandering in the Footsteps of Wordsworth

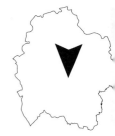

This jewel at the heart of the Lake District will have you reaching for your camera as you walk through breath taking scenery, steeped in history. Wandering the paths where Wordsworth composed his famous poems, you will circle the beautiful waters of Grasmere and Rydal Water, and experience first hand why Wordsworth called this ' the loveliest spot man hath ever found'

The start, in the delightful Grasmere Village, is outside the 13th century St Oswalds church where William Wordsworth is buried.

The Grasmere lakeshore footpath leads around the lake and through woodland to Loughrigg Terrace. Skimming stones and picnics are a lovely way to enjoy the lake. The view from Loughrigg terrace shows the lake district in all its glory, with an awe inspiring view of surrounding central Lakeland fells.

On to Rydal water, one of the lake districts smallest lakes, and an exploration of Rydal Cave, an old slate quarry developed towards end of the 19th century and closed in mid 1920s.

Crossing the river Rothay, Rydal is entered through Doras Field, a semi open woodland owned by the national trust. Wordsworth gave this land to his daughter Dora and he planted hundreds of daffodil bulbs in her memory when she died.

In Rydal two historical properties are open for exploration; Rydall Hall was built in the 16th Century and is now a place of retreat and a conference centre, with impressive gardens.

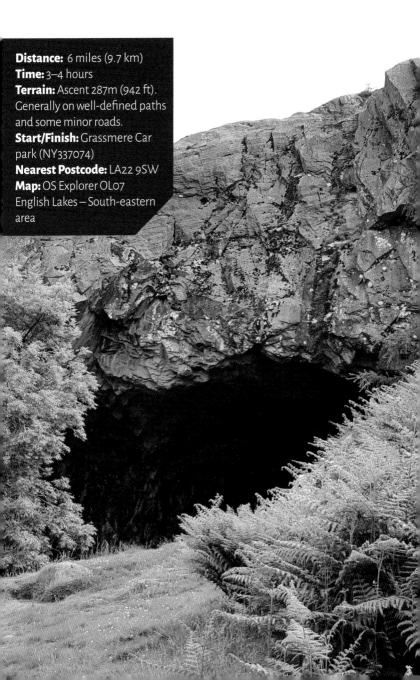

Distance: 6 miles (9.7 km)
Time: 3–4 hours
Terrain: Ascent 287m (942 ft).
Generally on well-defined paths
and some minor roads.
Start/Finish: Grassmere Car
park (NY337074)
Nearest Postcode: LA22 9SW
Map: OS Explorer OL07
English Lakes — South-eastern
area

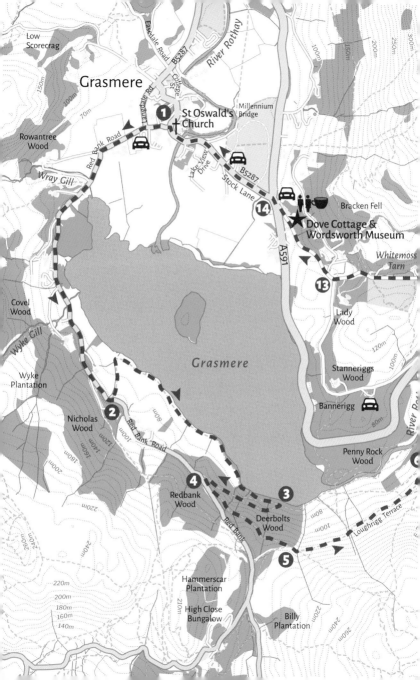

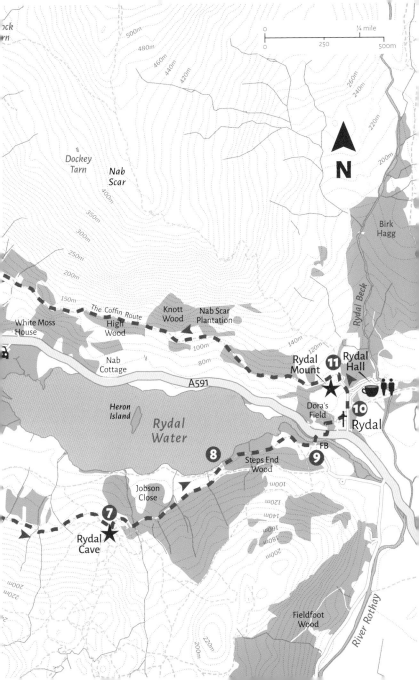

Rydal Mount was William Wordsworth's best loved family home and continues to be owned by the Wordsworth family.

The route back to Grasmere from Rydal follows the spookily named coffin route. This 'corpse path' was used by coffin bearers to take their dead to St Oswalds in Grasmere. The large stones on the path offer a good place to sit and reflect that in medieval times the coffin bearers would place the coffins on these stones to have a rest!

Approaching Grasmere village, the road passes Dove cottage lived in by Wordsworth in 1799, the adjacent Wordsworth Museum, and the Jerwood Centre an award-winning new building to house the collections of the Wordsworth Trust, opened in 2005.

1 Start outside the church. Cross the road and proceed along Red Bank road with the Garden Centre on the left. Continue along the road for 1.5 km (0.9 miles) until the Grasmere Lakeshore footpath is reached on the left.

2 Descend from the road to the lakeshore. Continue along the lakeshore and into Deerbolt Wood. 50 m before the lakeshore a track merges from the right.

3 Turn back sharp right and ascend to a cottage at a road.

4 Just before the road turn sharp left to continue on the track through the woods to reach a large gate.

5 Pass through the gate, over a small beck and onto the level Loughrigg Terrace bridleway until a junction of paths is reached.

6 Take the main path which descends with a wood on the left. After 50 m there is a gate into the wood. Take the footpath that starts opposite the gate and follow this for 600 m to Rydal Cave.

7 From the cave continue on the footpath as it zigzags down and on past more quarries on the right. After 500 m a lower path beside the lake comes into view. Take the small, initially stepped, path down to and across this lower path to enter Steps End wood at an old metal kissing-gate.

8 Follow this footpath through the wood, bearing left where the path splits, to a footbridge over the river.

9 Cross the bridge to reach the main road (A591). Turn right for 30 m and then cross the road and enter "Dora's Field" through a gate. Ascend on the path keeping right to enter the churchyard through a metal kissing gate. Take the path to the left of the church, through an arch, to reach Rydal Road by another gate.

10 Turn left and proceed up the road to reach the start of the "Coffin Route" bridleway on the left immediately after Rydal Mount. There is an option here to visit Rydal Hall – it's gardens and cafe on the right side of the road.

11 Proceed along the "Coffin Route" for 2 km (1.2 miles) until the end of a minor road is reached at Skater's Tarn.

12 Follow this road, keeping left at road junction with a seat, down to another road.

13 Turn right on the road and continue down to the main road (A591) passing a coffin stone and Dove Cottage on the right just before the main road.

14 Cross the main road at the roundabout and follow Stock Lane into Grasmere village and back to the start.

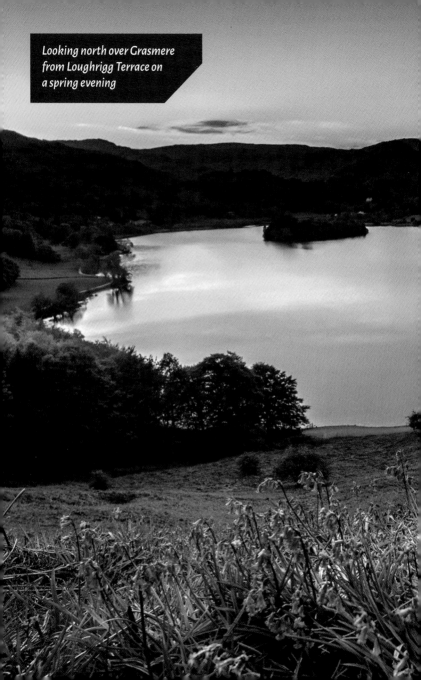
Looking north over Grasmere from Loughrigg Terrace on a spring evening

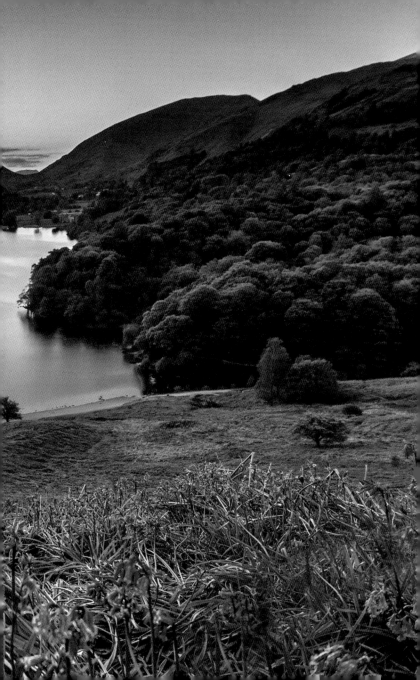

WALK 17
Langdale Valley

Enjoy some of the Lake District's most beautiful countryside, in the dramatic Langdale Valley.

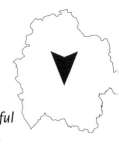

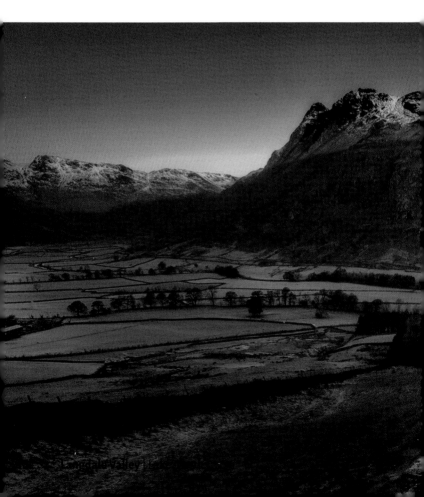

Langdale Valley Heras

This is a circular, clockwise walk starting from Elterwater National Trust Car Park – although you could just as easily start from one of the other car parks on the route. Elterwater and Old Dungeon Ghyll are served by the 516 bus from Kendal, Windermere and Ambleside.

The walk itself takes in woodland tracks, riverside paths and hillside trails, but there are plenty of inns, pubs and hotels to stop off in for refreshements, along the way.

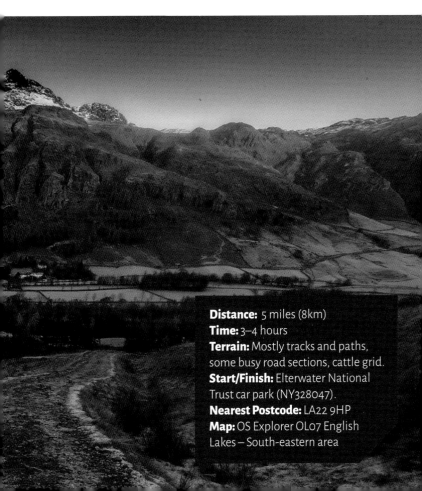

Distance: 5 miles (8km)
Time: 3–4 hours
Terrain: Mostly tracks and paths, some busy road sections, cattle grid.
Start/Finish: Elterwater National Trust car park (NY328047).
Nearest Postcode: LA22 9HP
Map: OS Explorer OL07 English Lakes – South-eastern area

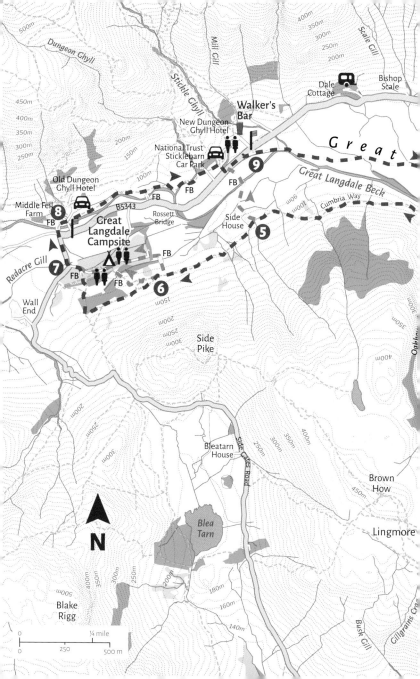

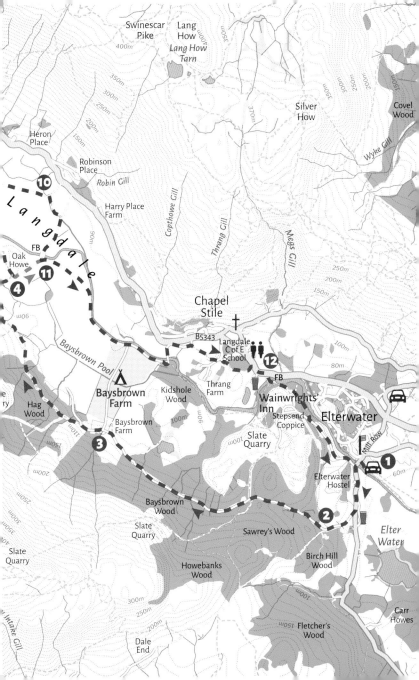

1 On leaving Elterwater car park turn left (Blue sign – Cycle Route 37 Coniston), pass the Elterwater Hostel and after 250 m turn right (Blue sign Coniston, challenging route). After 200 m keep right staying on the tarmac road (No Through Rd sign).

2 Follow the road to Baysbrown Farm where the tarmac ends.

3 Exit the farmyard keeping left, slightly uphill through a gate onto the bridleway to Oak Howe. After 300 m at a track junction bear right following finger post to Gt Langdale and road sign to Gt Langdale and Old Dungeon Ghyll (ODG). Continue on this bridleway for about ¾ mile.

4 Eventually, the bridleway takes a hard right turn and then comes a track junction by an interesting old barn with Oak Howe just beyond.

Optional: At this point the walk can be shortened by crossing the valley (heading to the right for about 200 m before picking up the returning path at point 11 (just before Great Langdale Beck).

Otherwise, to continue with the full walk, turn left at the cross track junction turn left following finger post sign for New Dungeon Ghyll (NDG). This is a section of the Cumbria Way – it can sometimes rough underfoot). The path now takes a large gentle bend to the the left over a distance of about a mile, before crossing a small clapper bridge and down a pitched path leading to Side House.

5 At Side House there is another opportunity to shorten the walk.

Optional: To cut back from here and avoid Old Dungeon Ghyll, simply follow the path to the right that cuts across the valley bottom (over a footbridge in about 250 m), to New Dungeon Ghyll.

Otherwise, to continue with the full walk, proceed slightly left up the field to a ladder stile over the wall. Continue across the next field to a second ladder stile, and step over low wall on the path above the NT campsite.

6 At this point you may wish to visit the campsite – drinks, snacks and WC. Otherwise continue on the field path to wood corner and on to meet a good track with kissing gate. Turn right, downhill through the woods, through several more kissing gates into the edge of the camp site. Note the old "slate gate gap" on the way which used wooden posts to create a barrier. A footbridge and yellow marker takes you left through the camper van hook up area and on to the road.

7 Turn right onto the road but at the post box leave the main road and go straight over the bridge before turning right, down the valley.

8 Stay on this path through two field gates. At a third gate pass through into a field onto a footpath signed Stickle Ghyll CP ½ mile. (To access ODG pub and CP go left at the third field gate). Continue across the fields, ignore the first bridge but cross the second bridge (yellow signs) over the field and into the Stickle Barn car park. Exit the car park via the access road to the main road B5343 and turn left.

9 Within 100 m or so cross the road near the bus stop onto the good track with the beck on right hand side. Stay on this track for about a mile until you get to a large track junction just below Harry Place farm.

10 Turn right, finger post Chapel Stile 2.25 miles and after 100 m turn right over bridge and cross the field on a very good path. Cross another bridge over Gt Langdale Beck.

11 Follow finger post sign to Chapel Stile. Pass below Baysbrown camp site on a concrete road – beware possible traffic. At the end of the concrete, turn left over cattle grid and bridge and follow road to holiday homes and track junction. Turn right (signed Village Centre) and at the junction by Langdale Primary School turn right again.

12 Turn right down the road past Wainright's Inn and follow the blue sign Elterwater ½ mile through a gate and over a bridge. This takes you onto the quarry road (beware large vehicles). Turn left down the quarry road to emerge in Elterwater with the CP just to your left.

WALK 18
Historic Hawkshead and Wray Castle

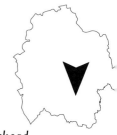

Discover the wealth of history around Hawkshead,
a viking settlement nestled in stunning scenery.

Shaped by the monasteries, developed by a characterful community and conserved by Beatrix Potter, Hawkshead has a rich tapestry of stories bursting to be told.

The walk starts at the grammar school, established by Edwin Sandy, Archbishop of York in 1585. It was attended by a young William Wordsworth in 1778.

Much of the history of the village comes from the church and the influence of Furness Abbey. Up until the turn of the 20th century the church was painted white which would have made it visible for miles around. Wordsworth referred to St Michaels and All Angels in 'The prelude': 'I saw the snow-white church upon her hill, Sit like a throned Lady, sending out a gracious look all over her domain'. The land around Hawkshead belonged to Furness Abbey and gifts of land were given to the tenants and named after them hence, 'Walker Ground', Keen Ground'. The Court House was originally built in the 13 Century and was administered by the monks who dealt with local disputes.

Beatrix Potter farmed around Hawkshead and left 4000 acres to the National Trust, ensuring the survival of the Lakeland landscape. The National Trust Beatrix Potter Gallery is now housed in the centre of Hawkshead.

In 1608 Hawkshead was awarded a market charter and was already the centre of the wool trade for North Lancashire.

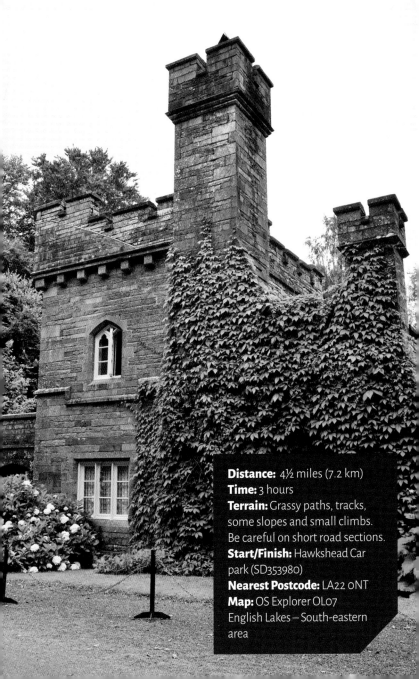

Distance: 4½ miles (7.2 km)
Time: 3 hours
Terrain: Grassy paths, tracks, some slopes and small climbs. Be careful on short road sections.
Start/Finish: Hawkshead Car park (SD353980)
Nearest Postcode: LA22 0NT
Map: OS Explorer OL07 English Lakes – South-eastern area

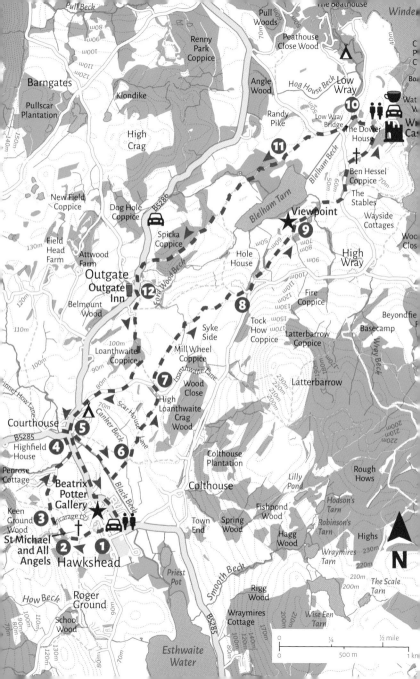

In addition to farming, many other trades flourished, with weavers, leather makers and tanning, builders, joiners and shoemakers, all making a living in and around the tiny streets now called Leather, Rag and Putty Street.

The section to Wray Castle walks over farmland and around Blelham Tarn, an important freshwater research site, to lake Windermere. Wray Castle is a Victorian gothic castle built in 1840 along with the neighbouring Wray Church. The house and grounds have belonged to the National Trust since 1929. Hardwicke Rawnsley was vicar of Wray church and became internationally known as one of the founders of the National Trust.

1 Start at the Old Grammar School and walk through the grounds to the churchyard, around the church. Leave by a metal gate to a 3-fingered signpost. Turn right following the sign headed Walker Ground.

2 Continue along the track to meet a small lane going up to Walker Ground Manor. Turn left and in 40m turn right through the gate.

3 Head away from the gate and after about 100 m there is a fence with a signpost to Tarn Hows. Pass over the wooden stile and walk ahead across the field, pass through a kissing gate, and continue ahead to meet the driveway to the Keene Ground complex. Turn right and follow this driveway down to the main road.

4 Turn left and take the main road for nearly 200 m to the 13 century Courthouse. Go back to the main road and carefully cross, going straight ahead into the field by Black Beck.

5 Take the gravelled path by the river bank, until the cross path is reached signposted Wray castle, then turn left. Continue along the track until the gate with the signpost to Wray Castle or Colthouse.

6 Turn left (signed Wray Castle) to reach Scar House Lane. Only head along this path for 30 m or so watching out for a gate to the right. Go through the gate on the footpath alongside a fence and continue along this path for about 300 m until you get to Loanthwaite Lane.

7 Turn left on the road for 100 m and then right down the side of the farm house. Follow the fence through fields and three gates.

8 Follow the National Trust sign to Wray through the Tock How farmyard and to the road. Turn left and the road drops down towards a white house. Head through the gateway past the house to cross a stone step-stile and continue along the track with stunning views of Blelham tarn and the Lakeland fells.

9 Continue along the track. The path leads to a small wood; enter through the gate and cross a bridge over the stream. Go up the hill and onto the road via a gate. Turn left on the road and follow it to the right at a junction past Wray vicarage to the entrance of Wray Castle.

10 After exploring the castle and lakeshore return to the main drive and walk to Dower House. Immediately after Dower House turn right along a bridleway signed Ambleside and Hawkshead; follow path downhill until a small lane is reached and turn left and walk to main road. Follow the road for about 50 m then cross road diagonally right to join bridleway/cycle route.

11 Follow the obvious path across a large field, into woodland and across the river with Blelham Tarn on the left. Look for a right hand path with a finger post to 'Outgate' and pass through the gate into Spicka Coppice. Walk up this uneven track to eventually arrive at the road and turn left to Outgate.

12 Immediately after passing Outgate Inn, turn left on to a footpath. Go through the gate and straight on through another gate across the field to the wood and follow the path to a lane. Turn right, then after about 300 m the lane joins the main road near to the Courthouse which was visited on the outward journey. Follow the main road back to the centre of Hawkshead village.

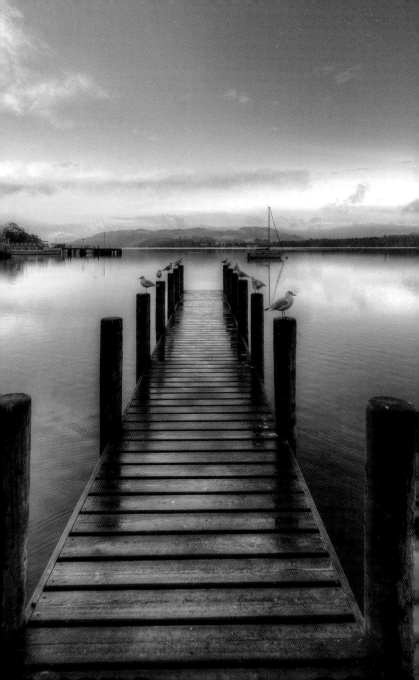

WALK 19
Orrest Head

Described by Alfred Wainwright as 'our first ascent in Lakeland' and 'a fitting finale, too, to a life made happy by fellwandering' – Orrest Head really is a fell walk for everyone.

There is a choice of routes to the summit, from wide paths, suitable for powered wheelchairs and prams, to rocky steps for those who prefer a bit of a challenge. The stunning 360 degree summit view is ample reward for the 30 minute approach and has inspired Wainwright and generations of walkers to further explore the beautiful Lakeland Fells.

Information panels at the start of the walk describe the choice of paths to the viewpoint. Choose the one which best suits your needs and enjoy exploring the lovely Elleray Wood as you meander up the hill to Orrest Head. The easiest path follows the route of an old Victorian carriage drive. It takes you past oak, birch, ash, beech, yew and sycamore trees, a walled garden and, in the spring, carpets of wild daffodils and bluebells.

Along the way, tantalising glimpses of the lake will whet your appetite for the view from the summit, while benches provide occassional rest points. The surprising appearance of a Gruffalo sculpture marks the halfway point.

Once the path leaves the wood for open pasture, you will come across a kissing gate flanked by memorial stones to Arthur Henry Heywood, the previous owner of Orrest Head and Elleray Wood. In 1902, his family gifted the land to Windermere for 'public walks'.

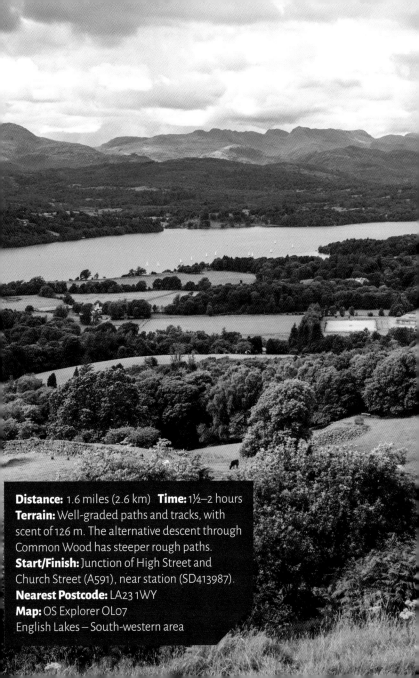

Distance: 1.6 miles (2.6 km)   **Time:** 1½–2 hours
Terrain: Well-graded paths and tracks, with scent of 126 m. The alternative descent through Common Wood has steeper rough paths.
Start/Finish: Junction of High Street and Church Street (A591), near station (SD413987).
Nearest Postcode: LA23 1WY
Map: OS Explorer OL07
English Lakes – South-western area

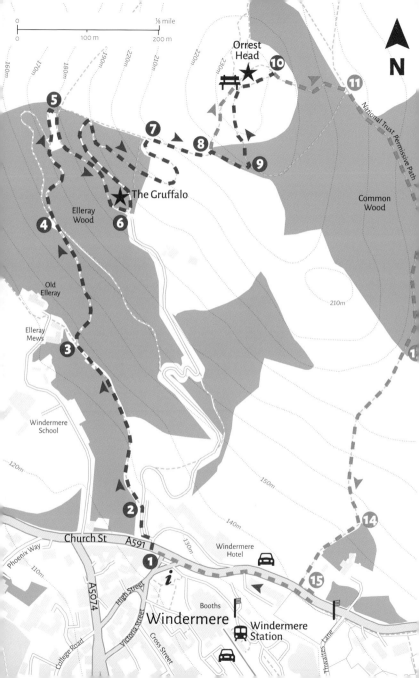

Orrest Head

10

11

5

7

8

9

National Trust Permissive Path

The Gruffalo

Elleray Wood

6

Common Wood

210m

4

Old Elleray

Elleray Mews

3

1

Windermere School

150m

2

140m

120m

130m

Church St   A591

1

Windermere Hotel

i

Phoenix Way

A5074

110m

High Street

Victoria Street

College Road

Cross Street

Booths

Windermere

Windermere Station

14

15

Thwaites Lane

0   100 m   200 m

0   ⅛ mile

N

The Orrest Head Compass crowns the summit. Have a seat to catch your breath and marvel at the view, then use the bench slats in this circular seating to take a bearing of the landmarks before you. A viewfinder nearby provides a Wainwright sketch of the Lakeland fells.

To return to Windermere, either retrace your steps or follow the route description down through Common Wood to enjoy more open views of the Lake.

1 Start opposite NatWest Bank at junction of High Street and Church Street (A591). Take the far left (tarmacked) track to Orrest Head. There is a map showing various colour-coded routes and the location of numbered signposts.

2 Keep left at the signpost for Orrest Head (signpost 1).

3 Turn right at the signpost (signpost 5) for Orrest Head and follow the walled track upwards into Elleray Wood to merge with another track (signpost 6).

4 Continue on the track with the wall to the left.

5 On a sharp bend in the track where a footpath leaves to the left (signpost 7) there is a choice of routes. The first route takes the steep stepped footpath beside the wall.

6 The easier option stays on the wide track to meet another track at the Gruffalo (signpost 8). Follow the track to the left and stay on the track as it sweeps gently uphill through the woods Both routes arrive at bench (signpost 10).

7 Continue a short distance, bearing right uphill until a kissing gate in the wall on the left (signpost 11).

8 Either pass through the gate and ascend steeply up steps to the summit (bypassing point 9) or continue on the track (passing signpost 12).

9 Turn left, through the wall gap, and follow the track to the summit (signpost 13).

10 Descend by retracing the uphill route.

Optional: An alternative descent route takes the National Trust Permissive Path through Common Wood. With the lake behind walk east to the right of the concrete seat with an inscription and take the righthand path to descend into Common Wood to a wall corner. Take care on the descent, as the path and tree roots can be slippery when wet.

11 Pass over the stone stile into a lane turning right to pass through a kissing gate into another wood on a narrow path.

12 Pass through a gap in a wall bearing right to follow a signpost for Windermere.

13 Leave the wood passing through a gate and descend in a field with a wall to the right to the start of a lane.

14 Temporarily leave the lane through the broken wall on the right to pass through a small gate, bypassing the locked gate in the lane. Follow the lane for a short distance to reach the main road (A591).

15 Turn left to cross the road at an island and then turn right on the pavement back to the start.

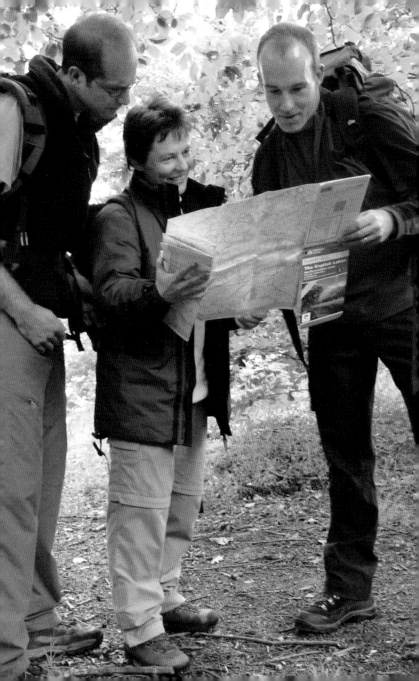

WALK 20
Cockshott Western Shore

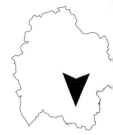

Bowness to Beatrix.

With glorious scenery you will want to applaud, this exploration of the central region of lake Windermere, exports you from the noisy bustle of Bowness – via the famous Windermere ferry – to the serene west shore and the solitude of Claife heights. The inspirational impact of Beatrix Potter can be seen across the landscape as you walk through wood, past tarn and over fell, and experience local historical influences on the way.

Cockshott point, an unassuming respite from the Bowness crowds, has history. It was the launching place for a Seaplane joyride in the early 1900s, and during the seventeenth century Civil War, Parliamentarians fired cannon from the shore at the Royalists on Belle Isle.

The Windermere ferry affords an excellent view of Belle Isle as it sails people, vehicles, horses and cycles across the lake. Belle Isle is the largest and only inhabited island on Windermere. There has been a ferry on the site for over 500 years, the earliest ferry being a rowing boat. The modern *Mallard* is pulled across by cables with a crossing taking about 10 minutes.

The west shore of Windermere is an easy amble along a wooded shoreline, with views of the Troutbeck fells and Bowness. The pebble beaches offer plenty of places to picnic, swim and watch the world go by on a sunny day.

Leaving the shore and walking through woodland over Claife heights to Far Sawrey brings the legacy of Beatrix Potter to life. Although best

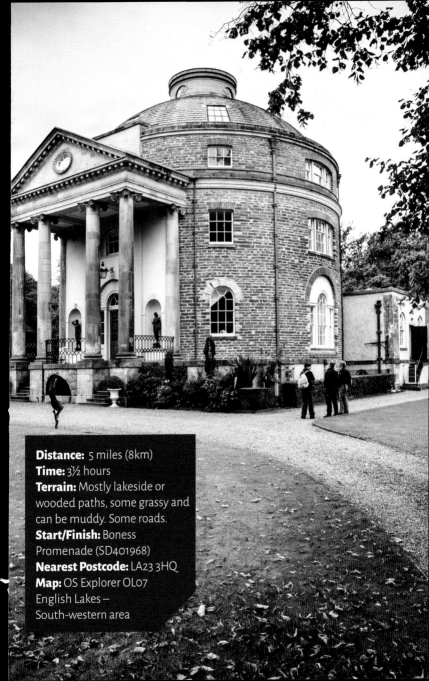

Distance: 5 miles (8km)
Time: 3½ hours
Terrain: Mostly lakeside or wooded paths, some grassy and can be muddy. Some roads.
Start/Finish: Boness Promenade (SD401968)
Nearest Postcode: LA23 3HQ
Map: OS Explorer OL07 English Lakes – South-western area

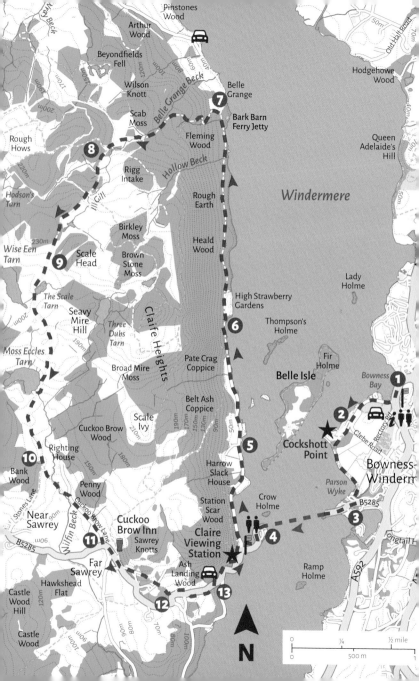

Pinstones
Wood

Arthur
Wood

Beyondfields
Fell

Wilson
Knott

Scab
Moss

Belle Grange Beck

Belle
Grange

⑦

Bark Barn
Ferry Jetty

Fleming
Wood

Hollow Beck

Rough
Earth

Heald
Wood

Hodgehowe
Wood

Queen
Adelaide's
Hill

Windermere

Rough
Hows

⑧

Hodson's
Tarn

Ill Gill

Rigg
Intake

Birkley
Moss

Wise Een
Tarn

⑨

Scale
Head

Brown
Stone
Moss

Claife Heights

High Strawberry
Gardens

Thompson's
Holme

Lady
Holme

The Scale
Tarn

Seavy
Mire
Hill

Three
Dubs
Tarn

⑥

Fir
Holme

Moss Eccles
Tarn

Broad Mire
Moss

Pate Crag
Coppice

Belle Isle

Bowness
Bay

①

Belt Ash
Coppice

②

Scale
Ivy

⑤

Harrow
Slack
House

Cockshott
Point

Crow
Holme

Glebe Road

Bowness-
Winderm

Cuckoo Brow
Wood

Righting
House

Penny
Wood

Station
Scar Wood

Parson
Wyke

B5285

⑩

Bank
Wood

Near
Sawrey

⑪

Cuckoo
Brow Inn

Sawrey
Knotts

Claire
Viewing
Station

④

③

Longtail H

Wilfin Beck

Far
Sawrey

Hawkshead
Flat

Castle
Wood
Hill

Ash
Landing
Wood

⑫

⑬

Ramp
Holme

A592

Castle
Wood

N

0   ¼   ½ mile

0   500 m

known for her childrens books she was passionate about conserving the landscape. She bought a number of farms and land, including Moss Eccles tarn which is said to have inspired the story of Jeremy Fisher, and where she spent many an hour fishing. She lived in Far Sawrey and when she died in 1943 left 4000 acres and 15 farms to the National Trust, ensuring the survival of the Lakeland landscape.

Dropping back to the ferry, enjoy a visit to Claife Station with its spectacular views. Dance with the echoes of the wealthy tourists of the 1830s/40s who enjoyed the panorama whilst dancing the night away at elegant parties held in the station.

The ferry will transport you back to your starting point.

1 From the ticket offices by the jetties follow the path around the shoreline keeping the lake on the right hand side.

2 Where the road bears left continue ahead, signed Hawkshead via Ferry ½ mile, passing through the gate at the entrance to Cockshott Point and follow the gravel path.

3 Turn right at a t-junction onto a broad track passing boatyards on the right to reach the road. Turn right onto the road down to the ferry.

4 Exit the ferry and follow the road for 150 m. Turn right through a gate opposite the bus stop, signed Claife Viewing Station ¼ mile. Follow the shoreline and pass through another gate. Turn right onto the public byway, signed Bark Barn 2 miles, following the lake shore.

5 Go through a gate to bypass the cattle grid onto the Claife Estate. Continue following the tarmac track along the shore. Go through another gate to by-pass the cattle grid. And continue along the side of the lake on the gravel track, signed Wray Castle Lodge 2½ miles.

6 At Strawberry Gardens continue straight ahead through the woods, signed Bark Barn 1 mile. Continue ahead past Bark Barn ferry jetty for 50 m to reach a path junction.

7 Turn left onto the path signed Hawkshead 3 mile and climb steadily keeping straight on where a path joins from the left. The path levels out and passes an information panel for Scab Moss. Continue ahead crossing a forest track and almost immediately bear left onto a bridleway signed Sawrey via Tarns.

8 Continue straight ahead at the first crossroads to reach a T-junction with a track. Bear right onto this track to reach a gate at the edge of the woodland.

9 Go through the gate and follow a good path past Wise Een Tarn on the right. Go through a gate and continue past Moss Eccles Tarn and through another gate to reach a fork in the track.

10 Bear left through a gate following the bridleway to Far Sawrey. and soon pass through another gate to by-pass a cattle grid. Continue and then bear right onto a tarmac driveway, pass through a gate to by-pass a cattle grid, continuing until a road is reached. Turn left along the road for 200 m passing Cuckoo Brow Inn on the left.

11 Bear left just past the phonebox/defibrillator on a footpath signed Ferry to Bowness. Pass through a metal kissing gate and continue ahead crossing a number of driveways to reach a wooden gate. Go through the gate and head downhill and through a wooden kissing gate following the signs to the ferry.

12 When the road is reached turn left for 100 m and at a road junction take the sheltered path on the right hand side signed to the ferry. At the end of the path cross the road and take the continuation of the sheltered path on the left hand side to the car park at Ash Landing.

13 Go through the car park and take the broad track signed Claife Viewing Station ¼ mile passing a low wooden barrier. Ascend the stone steps on the left hand side. At the top turn left to visit the viewing station. Return to the top of the steps and continue along the track signed Station Cottage & Courtyard ¼ mile. Pass through the courtyard to the road and almost immediate turn right through a gate to return to the ferry.

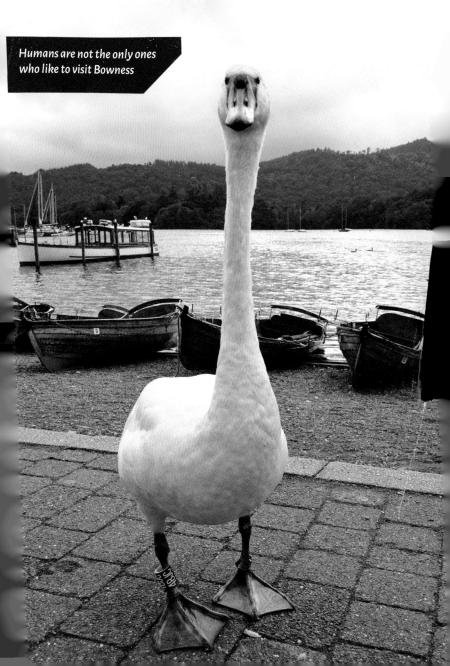

Humans are not the only ones who like to visit Bowness

Acknowledgements

Thanks to all of the photographers who allowed us to use their imagery in this book:

Page 6 © John Hodgson, page 12 © Keith Moore, page 19 © LDNPA, page 23 © Keith Moore, page 25 © John Hodgson, page 29 © David Askham/ Alamy Stock Photo, page 33 © John Morrison/ Alamy Stock Photo, page 37 © Andrew Locking, pages 40–41 © Joe Dunckley/ Shutterstock, page 43 © David Jarrott/Shutterstock, page 47 © Stephen Fleming/ Alamy Stock Photo, page 53 © Robbie Proctor/Shutterstock, page 57 © angus reid/Shutterstock, page 59 © LDNPA, page 63 © A D Harvey/Shutterstock, page 65 © Richard Bowden/Shutterstock, page 69 © Steve Heap/Shutterstock, page 73 © Fotimageon/Shutterstock, page 75 © Shen Stone/Shutterstock, page 79 © John Hodgson, page 81 © Kevin Standage/Shutterstock, page 85 © Rodney Hutchinson/ Shutterstock, page 87 © Andrew Roland/Shutterstock, page 90 © Keith Moore, page 93 © John Hodgson, page 97 © Keith Moore, pages 102–103 © LDNPA, pages 104–105 © LDNPA, page 111 © EQRoy/ Shutterstock, page 115 © EQRoy/Shutterstock, page 117 © Anna Mente/ Shutterstock, page 121 © LDNPA, page 123 © John Hodgson, page 127 © EQRoy/Shutterstock

Special thanks everyone who helped put this book together and especially to all the volunteers who helped check the routes:

Nicky Beeson, Tricia Brown, Andy Clifford, Mark Dalman, John Dennis, Catherine Dixon, Tony Edwards, Elaine Fisher, Barry Grayburn, Sally Minchom, Howard Simpson and Ian Verber

Maps © OpenStreetMap contributors
Contains OS data © Crown copyright [and database right] 2021.
Map creation: Cosmographics Ltd (www.cosmographics.co.uk).
Page design and layout: mapuccino (mapuccino.com.au).